W9-BVJ-611

ON PLUTO:
Inside the Mind of Alzheimer's

By Greg O'Brien

Foreword by Lisa Genova
Epilogue by David Shenk

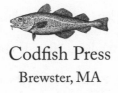

Codfish Press
Brewster, MA

© Greg O'Brien, Codfish Press, Brewster, Ma.

ISBN 978-0-9758502-1-3 hardcover
ISBN 978-0-9913401-0-1 paperback

Second Printing

Book design/page layout, Joe Gallante, Coysbrook Studio, Harwich, Ma.

Cover design: Brandy Polay

Printed by Paraclete Press, Brewster, Ma.

In Praise of *On Pluto: Inside the Mind of Alzheimer's*

"Told with extraordinary vulnerability, grace, humor, and profound insight, *On Pluto* is an intimate look inside the mind of Greg O'Brien, a journalist diagnosed with early-onset Alzheimer's. But the real gem of *On Pluto* lies in its unflinching look inside Greg's heart. If you're trying to understand what it feels like to live with Alzheimer's, and you are because you're reading these words, then you need to read this book." —**Lisa Genova, *New York Times* best selling author of *Still Alice***

"In *On Pluto*, Greg O'Brien has given us a priceless gift: an honest, funny, heartbreaking, and powerfully poignant look into the world of an Alzheimer's sufferer by a man who lives with it. Greg O'Brien is a brilliant observer and superb writer, and he is at the top of his game in this book. It's as if he has willingly dropped himself into a kind of mental tornado, so that he can tell us what he sees from inside. You have never read a book quite like it, and probably never will again." —**William Martin, *New York Times* best selling author of *Cape Cod, Back Bay,* and *The Lincoln Letter***

"Greg O'Brien writes with the consummate knowledge of a guide and the courage of a pioneer. In this important and transcendent book, he serves both roles as he folds back the veils of fear and traverses the treacherous territory of early-onset Alzheimer's. *On Pluto: Inside the Mind of Alzheimer's* glows with honesty, intelligence, and compassion, and, given the subject, is a surprisingly spirit-renewing book." —**Anne D. LeClaire, author of best selling *Listening Below The Noise, Leaving Eden,* and *The Lavender Hour***

"Most sufferers of early-onset Alzheimer's do their very best to hide it from everyone, sometimes even themselves. Greg O'Brien has chosen to look the beast in the eyes, and give us a candid, unflinching portrait of his family's tragic history of the disease, as well as his own determination to not go down without a fight." —**Steve James, producer of the short film** *"A Place Called Pluto"* **and considered among the most acclaimed documentary producers with noted works:** *Hoop Dreams, Life Itself, Stevie, The New Americans, The War Tapes, At the Death House Door,* **and** *The Interrupters*

"Alzheimer's messed with the wrong man. If there's anyone who can stand up to this awful disease with the right blend of eloquence, anger, and honesty, it is the defiant and profound Greg O'Brien. This book is a beacon of hope for anyone who can read or listen." —**David Shenk, author of** *The Forgetting,* **a** *New York Times* **best seller, and creator of** *Living With Alzheimer's* **film project**

"Greg O'Brien's daily movements now include, he tells us, periodic trips to Pluto, a dark and distant planet off the grid of enduring memory. But Greg's story of his life has mapped for us an inner space that is as light and present as Pluto is bleak and lonely. The courage of this book lies in the way that Greg speaks his peace into the dark. The hope of this book lies in the way that the dark, in the least expected of moments, seems to be listening to Greg, in inextinguishable love." —**Michael Verde, founder, Memory Bridge, The Foundation for Alzheimer's and Cultural Memory**

"Greg O'Brien takes us on a personal journey into Alzheimer's disease and marks the trail for others traveling this treacherous path. At once fighting and accepting his fate, he eloquently describes the delicate balance between living and dying with this mind-robbing disease. As his mind fails and his wisdom grows, he is teaching us to defy the popular notion that memory is everything." —**Daniel Kuhn, MSW, author of** *Alzheimer's Early Stages: First Steps for Family, Friends, and Caregivers*

"Never before have we been offered such a clear understanding of how Alzheimer's disease affects day-to-day perceptions. Greg O'Brien's first-hand account of his own disease process will force us all to rethink the way we deliver care, and is a must addition to the libraries of all professional and family caregivers." — **Suzanne Faith, RN psych, Clinical Director, Hope Dementia & Alzheimer's Services**

"As a clinician working daily with families and individuals dealing with Alzheimer's and dementia, the question we most often grapple with is how does one live well with the disease? Greg O'Brien's book, *On Pluto: Inside the Mind of Alzheimer's*, offers an answer rich in wit, courage, and a precision of detail that makes the book not only informative, but an extremely satisfying read. For the 5.4 million American families currently dealing with dementia, and for those of us who serve them, *On Pluto* is a critical and groundbreaking book. We are fortunate to have Greg's voice and spirit among us; he is a true American hero." —**Dr. Molly Perdue, PhD, Director of Family Services, Hope Health of Cape Cod**

"Greg O'Brien's personal battle against Alzheimer's is an everyman's fight; he is the quintessence of the lead character in the epic Alzheimer's novel, *Still Alice*. O'Brien, through faith, humor, and journalistic grit, is able, like a master artist, to paint a gripping, naked word picture of this progressive, chronic disease for which there is no cure—a sickness that will swamp a generation. O'Brien bluntly offers Baby Boomers and generations to come a riveting guide of how to live with Alzheimer's, rather than dying with it." —**Alisa M. Galazzi, co-founder of Dementia Care Academy, former Executive Director, Alzheimer's Services of Cape & Islands**

Contents

DEDICATION

To my mother, Virginia Brown O'Brien, whose
courageous battle with Alzheimer's taught me how to
stand firm in faith against a demon of a disease.

Romans 5:3-5—"We exalt in our tribulations, knowing
that tribulation brings about perseverance; and
perseverance, proven character; and proven character,
hope; and hope does not disappoint."

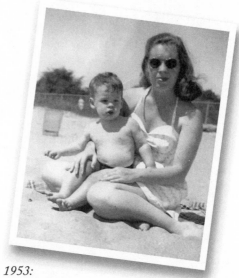

Age of innocence, 1953:
Virginia Loretta Brown O'Brien,
Rye Beach, Westchester County, NY, with son, Greg.

FOREWORD:

LISA GENOVA

Every story has a beginning, middle, and end. I met Greg O'Brien somewhere in the middle. I received an email from him the end of March 2011. He introduced himself as a journalist, a fellow Cape Codder, someone who knows my husband and his documentary film work, and a fan of *Still Alice*.

It was an email aimed to woo and impress me, and just as I was thinking this, I read:

"Don't be overly impressed by the articulation of this email. It took about two hours to write. Years ago, I would have written this in five minutes or less. But it was worth the time."

Like his mother and maternal grandfather before him, Greg had been diagnosed with early-onset Alzheimer's. He wanted to know if we could meet and talk. I get this kind of email a lot and do my best to offer an ear, encouragement, advice, and connections for further support. It's typically a sincere but brief relationship, most often limited to a few email exchanges. I had no idea when I agreed to meet Greg that he'd be on my mind pretty much every day since, that he'd become a close friend and personal hero.

Since I've known Greg, he's been fighting through the drifting fogs of dementia, determined to press on, drawing on everything he is—brilliant journalist, adoring and faithful family man, generous and lovable Irishman with a great sense of humor, masterful storyteller—to write *On Pluto*. Greg is the author of four Cape Cod-related books, and has won many prestigious awards for journalism over a 30-year career, but I believe this book is Greg's greatest achievement and contribution, not to the cure for Alzheimer's (at least not directly), but to our understanding of how to live and love in the presence of Alzheimer's.

In his own words, "While I have the facility to do so, I want to communicate to others, to those who will face this demon some day and those who love them, that with the proper medical direction, life strategies, faith, and humor one can prevail in the moment and lead a productive life for as long as possible."

Understanding the scientific pathology of Alzheimer's is critically important for improving diagnostic imaging, developing more effective treatments, and someday, discovering a cure. Understanding the science—the accumulation of amyloid and tau, identifying genetic risk factors, elucidating NMDA receptor regulation—is necessary and will take time and money.

But equally important to furthering research for a future cure is an understanding of the human experience of Alzheimer's now. What does it feel like to live with Alzheimer's? This kind of knowledge is also necessary, but it requires a different kind of investment. It takes courage and empathy.

We're all terrified of Alzheimer's. The fortress of fear, shame, stigma, alienation, and isolation that surrounds Alzheimer's today is not unlike what we saw with cancer 40 to 50 years ago. We didn't even say the word "cancer." Instead we called it "the big C" in hushed voices. But something changed. We began talking openly about cancer. We began wearing looped ribbons and walking to raise awareness and money, and as communities, we began rallying around our neighbors with cancer, offering dinners and carpools and support. We acknowledged the human experience of living with cancer. And now we have treatments for cancer. We have cancer survivors.

Right now, we have no Alzheimer's survivors. We need to find the courage to talk about Alzheimer's, to acknowledge not just the end of this disease, but also the beginning and the middle. We need to change the image of this disease, which tends to depict only an elderly person in end stage, "an empty shell," someone dying from Alzheimer's. Someone who is, perhaps, easier to ignore. This image excludes the millions of people LIVING with Alzheimer's, people newly diagnosed in their 40s, 50s, 60s, and 70s; people living somewhere in the beginning and the middle. People like Greg O'Brien.

What does it feel like to live with Alzheimer's? What does that image look like?

This is what Greg O'Brien so bravely, intimately, and beautifully shares with us. Recounting memories of his mother and grandfather, the day of his own diagnosis, symptoms of disorientation, stories of forgetting names and faces—even his wife, told with unflinching truth, grace, and humor, Greg shares with us what it feels like to live with Alzheimer's in the hope that we will better understand it. Understanding is the path to empathy. Empathy is the key to human connection.

Greg and I met a couple of years ago to talk about Alzheimer's. I expected to listen to this stranger, tell him what I knew, and help him out if I could. Then he'd be on his way, and I'd go back to my life without Greg O'Brien. Instead, I sat with a man so open and real, a man fighting to be present and live every single day to the fullest, with everything he's still got, a man who could find humor in the ugliest and scariest of moments. I was captivated, enamored, inspired. Surprised.

Since that day, Greg's Alzheimer's continues to advance, but the man I met more than two years ago is still here. He's tenacious, funny as hell, generous, incredibly smart, and brave. He's still open and real. He loves his family, his friends, and Cape Cod with a huge heart. He's a man I'm proud to call my friend.

Greg has told me many times that he believes his purpose is to share this story, that it might reach and improve the lives of millions of people traveling a similar journey.

I believe it will, Greg.

—Lisa Genova, PhD, *New York Times* **best selling author of** *Still Alice, Left Neglected,* **and** *Still Anthony*

PREFACE:

LIVING WITH ALZHEIMER'S

GREG O'BRIEN

"As I look back over a misspent youth, I find myself more and more convinced that I had more fun doing news reporting than any other enterprise. It really is the life of kings."—H.L. Mencken

Ascribe is nothing without good notes. For years I've taken detailed notes as an embedded reporter inside the mind of Alzheimer's, chronicling the progression of this monster disease. Ever since I knew that something was terribly wrong after a serious head injury had "unmasked" a disease in the making, my reporting instincts compelled me to document, to compile a blueprint of strategies, faith, and humor, a day-to-day focus on living with Alzheimer's, not dying with it—a hope that all is not lost when it appears to be.

Death comes to all. While in the natural, we have little rule over time and place, we can choose the attitude as we head through the tunnel to a brighter light. As Leonardo DaVinci observed in the 15th century: "While I thought that I was learning how to live, I have been learning how to die." Aren't we all, if we lift the thin veil of denial?

So, we press on in the shadows of role models. One of the most inspiring to me is a man called "Sweetness." He taught us legions on the gridiron about perseverance. The late Hall of Fame Chicago Bears legend, Walter Payton, nine times an All Pro, was one of the most prolific running backs in NFL history; he died too young at age 45 of cancer. Toward the end of his extraordinary career, a sports commentator declared on air in full reverence: "Walter Payton has run for more than nine miles!" To which his co-anchor replied intuitively, "Yes, and Payton did that getting knocked down every 4.6 yards, and getting back up again!"

If anyone has true grit in the fight against Alzheimer's, it is Glen Campbell. Diagnosed with the disease in 2011, he refused to retreat, courageously relying on his muscle memory as one of the nation's greatest songwriters and country and pop singers, teaching the rest of us along the way how to shine when the stage lights go dark. Campbell, while he could recall lyrics, launched his "Goodbye Tour" with three of his children joining him in his backup band. Sadly, in April 2014, it was reported that Campbell, at 78 still a man for all seasons in his inner soul, had become a patient at a long-term care facility.

Campbell was a lamppost to me earlier in life. I was drawn to his music on cross-country trips from New York to the University of Arizona where I attended school; his sweet, often raw and throaty voice, resonating from an eight-track tape cartridge, offered the verve to keep me focused and driving in my yellow Opel Kadett. His example today still keeps me focused and driving.

On these treks, I memorized almost every word of Campbell's Greatest Hits, produced in 1971, never forgetting to play repeatedly: "Wichita Lineman" as I crossed Kansas; "By the Time I Get To Phoenix," as I drove through the Petrified Forest in remote northeastern Arizona, often at 2 am with moonlight glistening off the semi-desert shrub steppes and colorful badlands; and "Gentle On My Mind" as I passed the graceful Santa Catalina Mountains, rising from the valley on the outskirts of Tucson. I can hear his voice now.

Award-winning filmmakers James Keach and Trevor Albert have eloquently captured the marvel of Campbell's music, his love of family, and his battle with Alzheimer's in a distinguished documentary, *Glen Campbell . . . I'll be me*. For anyone seeking to understand the journey of Alzheimer's and the endless solitary struggle of those afflicted "to be me," this Keach/Albert documentary is required viewing; it is edifying to the point of boundless wisdom. Campbell is a "Rocky with a guitar," Keach has said.

And then there's Pat Summitt, the legendary retired coach of the Tennessee women's basketball team, who told the *Knoxville News Sentinel* after announcing her diagnosis of early-onset Alzheimer's: "There's not going to be any pity party, and I'll make sure of that . . . Obviously, I realize I may have some limitations with this condition since there will be some good days and some bad days."

And so it is with chronic illness, good days and bad days. You get knocked down, you get back up. Again and again. You find a way to win—as New England Patriots Coach Bill Belichick would insist—on the playing field, on the job, in the home, or in a fight against cancer, heart disease, AIDS, Parkinson's, autism, depression, diabetes, dementia, or any number of vile illnesses. Lying down in football, as it is in wrestling, is a position of defeat. That's not a good place for any of us. As a famed billboard on Boston's Southeast Expressway proclaimed in the early '70s about Boston Bruin premier center Phil Esposito: "Jesus Saves. But Esposito scores on the rebound!"

My place today is with the disease early-onset Alzheimer's; it's a death in slow motion. A freeze frame at times. Alzheimer's and its predecessor, hardening of the arteries, stole my maternal grandfather, then my mother. And now it's coming for me.

Doctors tell me I'm working off a "cognitive reserve," a backup tank of inherited intellect that will carry me in cycles for years to come. They tell me to slow down, conserve the tank. It's lights out, they warn, when the tank goes dry, just as it was for my mother. In laymen's terms, the "right side" of my brain—the creative, sweet spot—is intact, for the most part, although the writing and communication process now takes exponentially longer. The left side, the area of the brain reserved for executive functions, judgment, balance, continence, short-term memory, financial analysis, and recognition of friends and colleagues is, at times, in a free fall. Doctors advise that I will likely write and communicate with declining articulation, until the lights dim, but other functions will continue to ebb. Daily exercise and writing are my succor, helping me reboot and reduce confusion. I try to stay locked in, as a missile is on target, but "locked in" likewise is a medical disorder in which an individual who cannot speak because of paralysis communicates through a blink of an eye. Some days, I find myself between definitions—using every available memory device and strategy, cerebral and handheld, to communicate.

All the darkness in the world, my mother taught me, cannot snuff out a single candle. I know that darkness. It's a place I call "Pluto," in allegorical terms, a reference from my early days as an investigative reporter when I went deep "off-the-record" with sources. "We're heading out to Pluto," I would say, "where no one can see you or can hear what is said."

The Pluto metaphor still works for me, more than ever, as I seek the peace of isolation and pursue the urge to drift out as Alzheimer's overcomes at intervals. Pluto is the perfect place to get lost. Formerly, the ninth planet about 3.1 billion miles from Earth, it is now relegated to "dwarf planet" status. Pluto's orbit, like Alzheimer's, is chaotic; its tiny size makes it sensitive to immeasurably small particles of the solar system, hard-to-predict factors that will gradually disrupt an orbit. Over the years, I've taken close family, colleagues, and clients "out to Pluto" to discuss off-record unmentionables of life in a place without oxygen. One day, like my grandfather and my mother, I won't return from this dark, icy place; when that happens, I want family and friends to know where I am.

The Irish like to say, "Never get mad, get even." And so, I'm getting even with Alzheimer's—not for me, but for my children, for you and your children, and for a generation of Baby Boomers, their families and loved ones, who face this demon prowling like Abaddon.

On Pluto: Inside the Mind of Alzheimer's is not a pity party or a misery memoir. It is an insider's guide, a generational road map of how to battle this cunning killer for as long as possible. To fight an enemy, one must study the enemy, and have working strategies in place. As the great ancient Chinese General Sun Tzu, assumed author of *The Art of War*, once counseled, "Tactics without strategy is the noise before defeat."

There is plenty of noise on the Alzheimer's front today, much defeat, and hardly enough funding for a cure. Not even close.

****

Alzheimer's, named for Dr. Aloysius "Alois" Alzheimer, who in 1906 first identified amyloid plaques and neurofibrillary tangles that rob the brain of identity, is the most common form of dementia—an umbrella term for irreversible cognitive collapse. Alzheimer's progresses slowly in stages, slaying neurons in the brain. The early stage is marked with increasing impairment of learning and short-term memory with some language challenges. The moderate stage is a progressive deterioration that leads to incapacity to perform certain common daily functions: short-term memory worsens, filter is lost, rage is intense, inability at times to recognize familiar places and people; some urinary and bowel incontinence; and at times, "illusionary misidentifications," which the layman, less politely, would term hallucinations.

I've entered the moderate stage, doctors say, but there is plenty of baseball left to play. The advanced stage—the stereotypical perception of Alzheimer's—is characterized by wandering and a complete shutdown of cognitive and body functions. Collectively, this slow demise can take up to 20 years or more once it's been diagnosed, and can begin ten or 15 years before diagnosis. With some, the progression, for reasons unknown, is far quicker.

This is not your grandfather's disease; it is fast becoming a disease of the young or young at heart. It's been said that Alzheimer's is like having a thin sliver of your brain shaved off every day.

Stephen King couldn't have devised a better plot.

Should you be frightened if you frequently forget where you put your keys? Maybe it's nothing, perhaps a "senior moment," or maybe it is the start of something. There is a clear distinction between forgetting where you parked your car and forgetting what your car looks like; forgetting where you put your glasses, and forgetting that you have glasses; getting lost on familiar roads because you've been daydreaming, and getting lost because your brain's capacity to store information is greatly diminished.

The numbers don't lie. They are numbing, and may be working against you, as the world's population grays. It's been said that, in 25 years, there will be two kinds of people in the world: those with Alzheimer's and those caring for someone with the disease. Consider this:*

- Alzheimer's is the sixth leading cause of death in the United States and the only such disease on the rise.

More than five million Americans have been diagnosed

*Alzheimer's Association *Alzheimer's Disease Facts and Figures.*
Accessed December 15, 2013. http://www.alz.org/alzheimers_disease_facts_and_fgures.asp

today with Alzheimer's or a related dementia and about
35 million people worldwide.

• In the next 36 years, just half a generation from now, the
number of individuals in the U.S. age 65 and older with
Alzheimer's disease is anticipated to nearly triple to a
projected 16 million, barring any medical breakthrough to
prevent, slow, or stop the disease. Worldwide, by 2050,
about 135 million are expected to have some form
of dementia.

• In the next 15 years, Alzheimer's is expected to exceed
cancer and heart disease sevenfold, and without a cure,
it will bankrupt Medicare. Soaring healthcare costs for
long-term care and hospice for people with Alzheimer's
and other dementias are projected to increase from $203
billion in 2013 to $1.1 trillion in 2050.

On Pluto: Inside the Mind of Alzheimer's is a story that might
be yours one day, or the story of a close friend or loved one;
please don't assume it won't. Some of the language within is
raw, full of rage, but real in its pain and fear. We can all learn
from Irish playwright George Bernard Shaw, who prophetically
observed, *"Life is no brief candle . . . It is a sort of splendid torch,
which I've got hold of for the moment, and I want to make it burn as
brightly as possible before handing it to future generations."*

All of us can assist future generations in the hand-off of a
cure for Alzheimer's, with a greater collective understanding of
the disease, more resources, and a worldwide commitment to
find a cure. My hope is that we all listen more. A pebble tossed
into a placid pond ripples far more than in roiling waters. In the
pages to follow, I offer a front-row seat into the mysteries of this
disease, an out-of-body experience on a trajectory to Pluto.

To understand this disease, one must step outside to see
inside.

ACKNOWLEDGMENTS

On Pluto: Inside the Mind of Alzheimer's has required more than six years of reporting, three years of writing, editing, and revisions, and more than two score of advisors, colleagues, family, and friends. This book would only be a concept without them. First of all, I would like to thank my wife of 37 years, Mary Catherine, and my children: Brendan, Colleen, and Conor, who sustain me and encouraged me to complete this work. Mary Catherine has been my mooring on this project; Brendan my mentor; Colleen my soul, who has opened many doors nationwide in the Alzheimer's community through her selfless volunteering; and Conor my rudder, keeping me grounded with his Celtic humor.

Secondly, I would like to thank close friend and celebrated author Lisa Genova, whose inspiration, encouragement, and guidance kept me on track, steadied me along the way, and pushed me when I needed to be pushed. Thank you! Her epic novel, *Still Alice*, has given voice and clarity beyond measure to those with Alzheimer's. She is a hero to the cause.

I am also grateful for a gifted team of advisors, writers, and editors who steered me along this serpentine path: my ever faithful right hand and director on this project, Alisa Galazzi, former executive director of the Alzheimer's Services of Cape Cod & the Islands; *New York Times* best selling authors Anne LeClaire and William Martin; editor Victoria Anderson; my personal physician Dr. Barry Conant, an inspiration to me; retired *Providence Journal* editorial page editor Robert Whitcomb, a former editor at *The Wall Street Journal* and *International Herald Tribune*; documentary producer George Pakenham, *Idle Threat*; film producer, author, and photographer Chris Seufert; author Ira Wood, founder of Leapfrog Press; Ken Sommer, former CEO of Visa International; Charlie Henderson; Terry and Jan Hoeschler and family; Mike Saint and Steve Shepherd; and the support of Sam Lorusso and Dave and Laura Peterson; Robert McGeorge; Ron Rudnick; Jim Botsford; Bill, Jonathan, and Betina Todd; Eric and Terri Guichet; Howard Hayes; Rick and Ella Leavitt; editorial advisors George Pakenham; as well as close friends Kristi Tyldesley, Paul and Leslie Durgin, Nancy O'Malley, Martha Hunter Henderson, Pam Hait, Mark Forest, Traci Longa; Scott Farmelant; and my nephew Kenny McGeorge for his soulful, never-say-die inspiration in his daily battle against advanced autism, a life lesson for me. Kenny keeps me fighting.

My sincere thanks also to close friends Ralph Branca, Patti Branca, and Mary Valentine; Dan and Kathleen Murphy; U.S. Senator Ed Markey, who has been a champion on Capitol Hill for the cause of Alzheimer's; *Cape Cod Today* publisher Walter Brooks; attorneys John Twohig, Jack Eiferman, and Teresa Foley of Goulston & Storrs of Boston, and Duane Landreth, Chris Ward, and Melanie O'Keefe of La Tanzi, Spaulding & Landreth on Cape Cod; author and CNBC television commentator Tom Casey; Ray Artigue, president of the Artigue Agency in Phoenix; Ed Lambert, WXTK-FM; Kevin O'Reilly, president of Creative Strategies & Communications; former *Arizona Republic* editorial writer Joel Nilsson and investigative reporter Chuck Kelly; writer John Lipman; *Cape Cod Times* Publisher Peter Meyer and editorial page editor William Mills, and Carol Dumas, editor of *The Cape Codder* for pressing me to persevere; and Vicky Bijur and Deborah Schneider.

Also, deep appreciation to Robert Kraft and Jonathan Kraft who taught me, through example, to find a way to win.

Much credit goes to legendary documentary director and producer Steve James *(Hoop Dreams, Stevie, Interrupters,* and *Life Itself)*; *New York Times* best selling author David Shenk *(The Forgetting, Alzheimer's: Portrait of an Epidemic, The Genius in All of Us,* and *Data Smog)*, a former advisor to the President's Council on Bioethics and a senior advisor to the Cure Alzheimer's Fund in Boston; and to Julia Pacetti of JMP Verdant Communications in Brooklyn. The Cure Alzheimer's Fund, in association with the MetLife Foundation, sponsored the production, with David Shenk as executive producer of four short films on the stages of Alzheimer's (livingwithalz.org), produced by world-class documentary producers. *A Place Called Pluto,* one of the films documenting my own family's journey in this disease, was produced by James. The films can be accessed on livingwithalz.org.

In addition, I would like to thank Adam Gamble, publisher of On Cape Publications for his steady direction in the production of this book; his skilled associate and author Mark Jasper; Mark Suchomel and Jeff Tegge of Legato Publishers Group, a division of the Perseus Books Group for outstanding effort distributing this book; Joe Gallante of Coy's Brook Studio for his impressive layout and design; and artist/graphic designer Brandy Polay for her stunning cover design. Polay knows firsthand of the struggle with Alzheimer's; she was a caregiver to her grandmother who died of the disease.

The Alzheimer's community on Cape Cod and the Islands was instrumental in guiding me and inspiring me along the process; among them: Molly Purdue, PhD, Director of Family Services, Hope Health of Cape Cod; Suzanne Faith, RN psych, Clinical Director, Hope Dementia & Alzheimer's Services; and Pat Collins, a key Hope Dementia & Alzheimer's Services associate. Hope Dementia & Alzheimer's Services of Cape Cod and the Islands (hopedementia.org) has been a lifeline in providing services to me and my family.

Speaking of family, in addition to my mother, I thank my father, Francis Xavier O'Brien, for pushing me, through his own example, to pursue a career in journalism. I thank my brothers and sisters: Maureen, Lauren, Justine, Paul, Bernadette, Tim, Andy, and deceased brothers Gerard and Martin for their love and hope at all celestial levels. I also thank Carl Maresca, Suzanne O'Brien, Peter O'Brien, Scott O'Brien, "Uncle" Mark O'Brien, Stephen and Melina Maresca, Lou McGeorge, Tommy and Barb McGeorge, Jerry Reardon and family, Larry O'Malley, Barbara Anne Newbury, Jeanne O'Brien, Sally O'Brien and family, and David Thompson. Also, I thank my 44 nieces and nephews; it might sound like a Gaelic cult, but family is the core of existence.

Also, special thanks to Ray Hunter; Tom and Kathleen Henze and family; Bob and Gretchen Kelly and family; Buzz Keenan; Buzz Keefe; Greg Keefe; Terry Sachi; Greg McGrath; Paul Hoffman; Brendan Bruder; special friend Marcia Calasio; Lisa Cooper; Terry Stewart; Dave Baby; Marty Hinds; Dave Ernest; Harry and Gena Bonsall; Adria Renke; Scott Burns; Jim Burns; and Tom and Debbie Woods.

Special recognition also to close friend and college buddy Pat Calihan, who died recently of dementia; to his devoted wife, Becky, and all of Pat's family. Pat, we will never forget you. Promise!

Finally, I thank friends and colleagues for their love and support, in no particular order: Peter, Aaron, and Matt Polhemus, and Francie Joseph; Jess Ritchie; Augusta Hixon; Bobby and Susan Norton; Tom and Peg Ryan; John and Katie Piekarski; Matt Everett; Tim and Maggie Everett; Mark St. John; Billy and Nancy St. John; Tony and Karen Keating; Jimmy and Debbie Dianni; Vinny and Kim Dempsey; Joe and Cathy Lewis of Joe's Beach Road Bar & Grille in East Orleans for their ongoing support; John Murphy and his family of the Land Ho! in Orleans; the gang at Mahoney's; close friends and supporters Dick and Nancy Koch; Charlie and Cindy Sumner; Dana and Gayle Conduit; Mark and Anne Ohrenberger; Uncle Cody Morrow, Tim Whelan, and John Terrio; Cape Cod Museum of Natural History Executive Director Bob Dwyer; Anne Saint; Frank Andrews; Pat Fox; Ricky Weeks; Frank and Carolyn Dranginis; Mike Gradone; Mark Mathison; Brian Kavanaugh; Geoff and Rebecca Smith; Vern and Missy Smith; Barry, Nancy, and Kristin Souder; Barbara and Matt Losordo; Pastor Doug Scalise; *The Martha's Vineyard Times* editor Doug Cabral; Eileen and Jeff Smith; Paul and Mitzi Daley; Donald and Jack Shea; Bill O'Brien; Joe Penney; Sarah Alger; Wally Steinkrauss; Deb Farr; Tim Mahoney; Dave Taglianetti; Randy Hart; Mike Ford; Jeff Ford; Rob Chamberlain; Steve Boyson; Lynda Walsh; Debbie Stewart; Joanne and Len Hensas; Melissa and Nathaniel Philbrick; Linda Edson; Linda Williams; Nat Lowell; Rick Turer; Barry and Joanne Powers; Sean Summers; producer Trevor Albert, and director/producer James Keach.

In reading this litany beforehand, my brother-in-law Carl joked, "*Really!* You could have included the Red Chinese and the Bolsheviks." Well, it takes a village with Alzheimer's.

In closing, I thank retired U.S. Supreme Court Justice Sandra Day O'Connor, whose husband, John, died of Alzheimer's. Justice O'Connor instructed me many years ago in the art of court reporting when I was a cub reporter at *The Arizona Republic* and she was a Maricopa County Superior Court judge. Justice O'Connor has been an enduring inspiration for families battling Alzheimer's.

Greg O'Brien

ON PLUTO:
Inside the Mind of Alzheimer's

1

A Place of Recall

THE WIND HAS SHIFTED ON CAPE COD. A RUSTED IRON COD on the weathervane at the gable end of the barn is pointing southwest, a warning of foul weather fast approaching from the nor'east. The weathered New England cedar shingles at a precise nine-inch pitch are wet with a fine mist. Near a side door, framed by lobster buoys washed up on the shoreline, a simple white dory window box is filled with colorful perennials. The barn has the feel of a dune shack, a writer's retreat at the end of a barrier beach—all of it natural, a reflection of the man and his memories snug within.

The door is open, revealing a time capsule of newspaper and magazine clippings, shelves of books, photos of the renowned, the infamous, and other memorabilia. I am innately connected to this man within and to his memories. In his early 60s, he is well kept, the product of running four miles a day; his horn-rimmed glasses and long tufts of graying hair evoke the look of a college professor. He strikes me as a bit of a prick, yet engaging. I know him, yet I can't relate in the moment. He's not the person I remember.

"Memory is deceptive, colored by today's events," Albert Einstein once observed.

Today's events are a flash for me, fully an out-of-body encounter, a flood of disconnected synapses, as I discern a flickering picture as if maneuvering rabbit ears on a vintage black-and-white TV, trying to get the focus just right. The human brain, a fragile organ that inaugurates connectivity the first week *in utero*, contains 100 billion neurons—16 billion times the number of people on Earth—with each neuron igniting more than 10,000 synaptic connections to other neurons, totaling more than a trillion connections that store memories. If your brain functioned like a digital video recorder, it could hold more than three million hours of TV shows, enough video storage for 300 years. Not bad for a mass the size of an average head of cabbage, with the encoding, storage, and retrieval capacity to determine, on a good day, how many angels can dance on the head of a pin.

So, why can't I get a clear picture today? The image is out of focus. When I look through this prism of an altered state, the picture is muddled. I press on for affirmation.

The man is the essence of a Baby Boomer—an over-achiever, an individual of purpose, gregarious, the oldest boy in an Irish Catholic family of ten, a father of three, husband of a virtuous wife for 37 years, the patriarchal uncle to 44 neices and nephews, and a man who always thought, until now, that better days lay ahead. That's the way it is with Boomers, the invincible generation—sons and daughters of the Greatest Generation whose grandparents endured World War I, and whose parents then survived the Great Depression and World War II, perhaps the last world conflagration until Armageddon. These Boomers, a record 75 million of them born between 1946 and 1964, first played by the rules, then broke the rules, then made new rules. Boomers grew up in a time when we thought shit didn't happen. I look to the walls to connect the dots. The writer within grew up in the '50s, formative years when Einstein was still thinking, Hemingway was still writing, and Sinatra was still crooning. Like all Boomers of the day, the man's early life reflects history: the long, fading shadow of Franklin Delano Roosevelt; the dropping of hellish atomic bombs on Hiroshima and Nagasaki; the Korean War; the election of presidents Dwight Eisenhower, John F. Kennedy, Lyndon B. Johnson, Richard Nixon, and all the baggage; the apocalyptic Cuban Missile Crisis; the Vietnam War; Woodstock; the birth of free love; and the death of innocence. It was a revolutionary time that spanned perhaps more cultural shifts than any other generation with writers, artists, and musicians who still define this country's political, secular, and artistic persona.

Isn't he a bit like you and me?

Looking around a room, one can learn legions from what's displayed on the walls. They paint "word pictures." Everywhere, there are historical, framed front-page stories and magazine covers from *The New York Times*, *The New Yorker*, *Washington Post*, the *Daily News*, the *Los Angeles Times*, the old *Boston Herald Traveler*, *Boston Record*, and one from the *Yarmouth Register*, dated July 12, 1861, reporting Abraham Lincoln's declaration to Congress of the Civil War. The office is a news museum of sorts, with news clippings of the firing on Fort Sumter, JFK's assassination, Nixon's resignation, Anwar Sadat's murder, the shooting of Pope John Paul II, the Shuttle explosion, the 9/11 attacks on the World Trade Center and Pentagon, and much more. In a corner is a frayed copy of the July 21, 1969 *Burlington Free Press* announcing that man has walked on the moon. Below the fold, toward the bottom of the page, is a photo of a 1968 Oldsmobile Delmont 88 that took a horrible turn for the worse into history off a narrow dike bridge on Martha's Vineyard. The caption directs readers to an inside story, the luck of the tragic Irish: Ted Kennedy's "Chappaquiddick incident," the death of Mary Jo Kopechne, buried on page six.

On the walls are news reports and magazine stories the man wrote years ago for publications—stories on Tip O'Neill, Jimmy Carter, the Kennedy family, Bill Clinton, the federal court system, political corruption, and investigative stories on the mafia. On a wicker chair nearby is a profile of a former Phoenix Superior Court judge, who in the late '70s mentored him at *The Arizona Republic* in the art of court reporting—Sandra Day O'Connor. Years later, President Ronald Reagan appointed the Stanford Law School graduate who grew up on an Arizona cattle ranch as the nation's first woman Supreme Court Justice. Judge O'Connor had urged her student repeatedly before leaving for Washington to keep asking questions.

"Keep at it until you get the answers!" she counseled.

And he does today.

Everything in this room tells a story, purposefully arranged in almost chronological order, as if to remind, almost reassure, its occupant of a timeline, a collective long-term memory, the hard drive of one's life, the answers—from historic events, to family photos, to memorabilia. In a curious contradiction, there's a hint of eclectic New York and Boston family roots, which clash over sports: framed headlines of the New England Patriots, Red Sox, Boston Celtics, and Boston Bruins, alongside classic black and white photos of a young Mickey Mantle, Yogi Berra, Joe DiMaggio, and Lou Gehrig. On a shelf below, a 1917 photograph of a sullen Babe Ruth in a Boston Red Sox uniform stares out blankly. There is a quote of Ruth's below it: "Never let the fear of striking out get in your way."

Curiously enough, tacked to an adjacent wall is a tale, author unknown, of an Irishman's dying wish with two strikes against him.

His Irish friends relate:

> *An elderly gentleman lay dying in bed. While suffering the agonies of a pending death, he suddenly smelled the aroma of his favorite chocolate chip cookies, wafting up the stairs. He gathered his remaining strength and lifted himself in the bed. Leaning against the wall, he slowly made his way out of the bedroom and with even greater effort, gripping the railing with both hands, he crawled downstairs. With labored breath, he leaned against the door-frame and gazed into the kitchen. Were it not for death's agony, he would have thought himself already in Heaven for there spread out on wax paper on the kitchen table were literally hundreds of his favorite chocolate chip cookies.*
>
> *Was the elderly Irishman in Heaven or was it one final act of heroic love from his Irish wife of 60 years, seeing to it that he left this world a happy man?*
>
> *Mustering one great final effort, he threw himself towards the table, landing on his knees in a rumpled posture. His parched lips parted; the wondrous taste of the cookie was already in his mouth, seemingly bringing him back to life.*
>
> *The aging and withered hand trembled on its way to a cookie on the edge of the table when he was suddenly smacked with a spatula by his wife ...*
>
> *Fuck off, they're for the funeral!*

There will be no funeral today, only an epiphany of what's to come, and with the luck of the Irish, maybe a few steaming hot chocolate chip cookies, as denial gradually gives way, over time, to reality. Stephen Stills had it right: "Love the one you're with."

I do.

For I must.

For this man is me.

2

MR. POTATO HEAD

ASEA OF SPRING DANDELIONS OUTSIDE THE BARN IS LEANING toward the bay in a stiff wind, a wave of yellow. They capture my attention. I am drawn to the cluster. The dandelion—a French derivative for "*dent de lion*," the tooth of a lion, with its sharp yellow leaves and believed to date back 30 million years— is born as a flower, becomes a weed, dies slowly from the head down; then its white, fluffy seeds, gentle blowballs, genetically identical to the parent plant, blow away to pollinate the world.

And so it is with Alzheimer's.

Ralph Waldo Emerson wrote in his essay *Fortune of the Republic*, "What is a weed? A plant whose virtues have not yet been discovered." Perhaps Emerson, who succumbed to Alzheimer's-like symptoms, was contemplating the dandelion—a free spirit of a plant, a symbol of courage and hope, with relevance in medicine, legend, and in Christianity. In medieval times, the dandelion, a bitter herb, was a symbol for the crucifixion of Christ. The virtue of Alzheimer's is a hope for redemption—not here for now, but beyond.

Sitting alone in my office, deep in thought, looking out over an acre of overgrown lawn, sprinkled with dandelions, and surrounded inside by the hard copy of long-term memory, a place where confusion gives way to clarity and humor resurrects, I remember the yarn of the septuagenarian who reluctantly arranged a medical exam after years of denial:

"I have some bad news for you," the doctor says after a battery of tests. *"You have cancer!"*

"That's dreadful," the man replies.

"It gets worse," the doctor notes.

"You have Alzheimer's!"

The man pauses to collect his thoughts, then says with full confidence, *"Thank God, I don't have cancer!"*

I laugh, but it's more an enigma than a joke.

Some inherit stock portfolios and buckets of cash. Others, hand-me-downs. I've inherited my folks' medical records: my late father, Francis Xavier O'Brien, a mulish second-generation Irish American and a Bronx boy, had prostate cancer, complicated by critical circulation disease and an onslaught in final days of dementia; my mother, Virginia Brown O'Brien, with second-generation Irish roots as well, the hero of my life, died of Alzheimer's in a bruising, knockdown prizefight of a battle, as her father had decades earlier.

I have been diagnosed with both —cancer andAlzheimer's.

I've declined cancer treatment for now, on grounds that no one by choice wants to go to a nursing home. I saw what Alzheimer's robbed from my grandfather and my mother, and learned earlier in life about "exit strategies" from seasoned venture capitalists in New York and Boston. Alzheimer's, to me, is far more distressing than my cancer. I'm looking now for an exit strategy.

You can't remove a brain.

Daily, I return to my office on the Cape in search of a past that has more relevance to me than the present or a future. There is great peace here among the elements of history, humor, and faith—cornerstones in my life. I look for strength from mentors, past and present, referenced in various clips and photos on the walls: celebrated country editors like the late Malcolm Hobbs of *The Cape Codder*, a surrogate father figure: the distinguished Henry Beetle Hough of the *Martha's Vineyard Gazette*, and my late neighbor John Hay, considered among the nation's finest nature writers, on par with Henry David Thoreau. Hay was a man who could paint brilliant word pictures with the stroke of a typewriter key as a master does with a brush. I was blessed in spending time with them, absorbing like a sea sponge as they taught me to write. They all have become an enduring part of what I believe a good writer, a persevering individual, ought to be. Perseverance separates the artist from the dabbler, editor Hobbs once told me. So it is with life; you press on.

Near my writing desk is a copy of the best seller, *The Perfect Storm*, known in these parts as the Halloween Nor'easter of 1991. I first met author Sebastian Junger as a young man when he was a budding scribbler, soon to be star, and I was an editor at *The Cape Codder*, instructing the freelancer in the art of reporting, letting a good story tell itself. Junger, an excellent student with extraordinary drive, excelled beyond all expectation. I find myself today in the midst of my own perfect storm—a rogue wave of fear, perhaps a life unfulfilled.

On a bookcase in the corner are photographs of my children—Brendan, Colleen, and Conor, and my wife Mary Catherine—all reminders of a past and a fleeting present. There is a recent precious photograph taken by Colleen at an Alzheimer's fundraising marathon that she ran in Boston. The photo is of a pure white running cap alongside two purple wrist bands, the symbolic color of the battle against Alzheimer's, all arranged on a stark linen table cloth. She wore them in the race. The cap is inscribed, "Dad, this is for you."

****

Dementia runs in my family, practically gallops on some branches of the family tree. My maternal grandfather, George Brown, died decades ago of "hardening of the arteries," a precursor for Alzheimer's, now considered a code word for Alzheimer's or vascular dementia. I had a chilling front-row seat as a child, and later, head-on with my mother's slow progression of a death in slow motion. My dad, in the waning months of a complicated medical history, was also diagnosed with dementia, and his only brother, my uncle, now suffers from a variant of Alzheimer's. The images are piercing.

In 2009, I was diagnosed with early-onset Alzheimer's, several years after first experiencing early symptoms and after a horrific head injury sustained years earlier in a bicycle accident that doctors say "unmasked" a disease in the making. Dumbass that I was, still am, I wasn't wearing a helmet at the time. Repeated clinical tests, an MRI, and a brain scan confirmed the diagnosis. The brain (SPECT) scan revealed "a large deficit involving the temporal parietal and also occipital lobes bilaterally," as noted in the blunt 80 pages of my medical records. That's code for pack your bags. Another test revealed that I carry a gene called ApoE4. Present in about 14 percent of the population and implicated in Alzheimer's, ApoE4 is a known genetic risk for the disease.

Inheritance indeed is a mixed bag. Doctors tell me that I'm working off a "cognitive reserve," a reservoir of inherited intellect that will carry me in cycles for years to come. They tell me to slow down, conserve the tank. I'm not sure how much reserve remains; I guess I'll find out how smart my mother was. I'm hoping she was a genius. The brain I inherited is like an old Porsche engine. It has to crank at high speeds, or it sputters. When I run out of gas some day, I hope I pull off the road to a place with a water view. For now, I keep driving, foot to the floor.

I strive to keep the focus today on *living* with Alzheimer's, not dying with it.

But the view within is out of sync many days. The "right side" of my brain—the creative sweet spot—is mostly intact, although the writing and communication process now takes much longer. The left side, reserved for judgment, executive functions, and financial analysis, is in a free fall on bad days. Doctors advise that I will likely write and communicate, with diminishing articulation, until the lights go out, as other functions continue to wane, an idiot-savant syndrone, I suppose.

"Plan for it," they have advised me.

But as the great Bambino once said, "You can't beat the person who won't give up."

These demons, I keep telling myself, *don't know who they're fucking with!*

Years ago, I thought I was Clark Kent, but today I feel more like a baffled Jimmy Olsen. And on days of muddle, more like Mr. Magoo, the wispy cartoon character, created in 1949, who couldn't see straight, exacerbated by his stubbornness to acknowledge a problem, or like Mr. Potato Head, with the wacky pushpins and all. The genius of Brooklyn-born investor George Lerner in the early 50s, the original Mr. Potato Head sold for 98 cents, was the first toy ever advertised on television, and came with pushpin plastic hands, feet, ears, two mouths, two pairs of eyes, four noses, three hats, eyeglasses, a pipe, and eight felt pieces resembling facial hair. Fifty years ago, Hasbro provided a plastic potato body, given complaints of rotting vegetables.

I think of myself now as Mr. Potato Head with a rotting head and stick-on body parts, depending on my mood and the brain's diminishing ability to function.

Before the onset of Alzheimer's, I thought of my brain as a large depository, a dumping ground of sorts, a large storage bin for stashing a cornucopia of politics, current events, sports, trivia, and points of view that nobody really cares about but me. In

Alzheimer's, the brain atrophies; it shrinks radically, a shrinkage of brain tissue. And I always thought shrinkage was what happened to guys after a dip in a cold ocean.

"Getting old ain't for sissies," Bette Davis once opined. She was spot on. We all need to put on our big boy and big girl pants.

****

Daily medications serve to keep my engine in tune and slow a progression of the disease: 23 milligrams daily of Aricept, the commonly prescribed Alzheimer's medication, the legal limit; 20 milligrams of Namenda in a combined therapy that serves to reboot the brain; 50 milligrams of Trazodone to help me sleep; and 20 milligrams of Celexa (Citalopram) to help control the rage on days when I hurl the phone across the room, a perfect strike to the sink, because in the moment I can't remember how to dial, or when I smash the lawn sprinkler against an oak tree in the backyard because I can't recall how it works, or when I push open the flaming hot glass door to the family room wood stove barehanded to stoke the fire just because I thought it was a good idea until the skin melts in a third-degree burn, or simply when I cry privately, the tears of a little boy, because I fear that I'm alone, nobody cares, and the innings are starting to fade.

Hey, I'm not stupid, nor are others with Alzheimer's; we just have a disease.

But on particularly down days, in between moments of focus, I feel a bit like a svelte stand-in for Curly Howard of The Three Stooges, lots of running in circles—"nyuk-nyuk-nyuk … woob-woob-woob!" Alzheimer's is a sickness that runs in circles or meanders for an eventual kill. It's analogous to the prototypical arcade game Pac-Man in which a pie-faced yellow icon navigates a maze of challenges, eating Pac-dots to get to the next level. While the iconic video game was designed to have no ending, there are no "power pellets" in Alzheimer's to consume the enemies of ghosts, goblins, and monsters, as this Pac-Man in slow motion consumes brain cells, one by one.

Game over!

"You're a pioneer," a counselor once urged me in a men's early-onset Alzheimer's support group, speaking before a gathering of lawyers, engineers, architects, and a minister—all diagnosed with the disease, and individuals as accomplished as one would find anywhere. "Take good notes," he urged us.

I have.

Having witnessed the demise of family members, seen the anguish firsthand inside nursing homes, felt the disconnect of dementia in intimate terms, I've overcome a reticence to speak out. There was a time when I worried about what family, friends, colleagues, and clients would think or say. No longer. I suppose one could say that I'm outing myself now. Gore Vidal once observed, "Style is knowing who you are, what you want to say, and not giving a damn."

I don't give a damn, if that's what it takes to get the word out.

As any writer knows, solid reporting follows a stock of knowledge. So, I've studied the brain to the extent that I can and have learned, over time, that it is the most energy-consuming part of the body; it represents about two percent of the body's weight, but has the raw computer power of more than 16 billion times the number of people on Earth. Without sufficient brain power, some suggest, we're like astronauts on a space walk whose lifeline has just been cut. We drift to the ends of the universe. Out beyond, to Pluto.

Boomers will drift, facing an unimaginable epidemic of Alzheimer's and related dementias, in projected numbers seven times greater than cancer or heart disease, whose critical research and funding starkly outpaces Alzheimer's tenfold. There are an estimated 35 million people worldwide today diagnosed with Alzheimer's or a related dementia, an estimated five million in the U.S. afflicted with Alzheimer's, and predictions of up to 13.8 million Americans diagnosed with the disease by 2050.*

Researchers suggest new ways of combating the disease. Alzheimer's in the making must be stopped long before it damages the brain, doctors say. Research shows that once an individual begins to lose synapse (the brain structure allowing a neuron, a nerve cell, to pass an electrical or chemical signal to another cell), and once neurons are lost, the brain cannot recover. Alzheimer's starts long before symptoms are apparent to others, perhaps ten or more years earlier, and if diagnosed early and treated with medications before loss of synapse, the progression may be slowed, although it cannot be stopped, as doctors are learning.

Part of living with Alzheimer's and slowing the progression is in the daily training regimen to accelerate synapse. Consider the jaggy dendrite we learned about in high school biology—a spine or tree-like projection of a neuron that passes signals to other brain cells. Exercising the brain, experts say, builds new dendrites, pathways that create alternate routes for synapse that can help one function with Alzheimer's for longer periods, while other neurons are dying off. In short, I believe, one can re-circuit the brain to receive and transmit information, staving off, for a time, some of the more horrific symptoms of this disease. But in the end, the neurons go dead.

This is the place I find myself today, pushing back daily against a loss of synapse that is progressing, as neurons go dead. The challenge with public perception of Alzheimer's is that few want to embrace the disease, take it seriously, at least not until a family member or close friend is found in a nursing home sleeping in urine and talking to the walls. Public awareness of this disease, a balance between science, medicine, and faith, needs to change dramatically in anticipation of an Alzheimer's epidemic for Baby Boomers and others to come. In a snapshot, Alzheimer's is not the stereotypical end stage; it is the journey from the diagnosis to the grave.

There is an upside: you can get out of jury duty in a New York minute!

****

Does loss of brain function render loss of self; can we thrive in spiritual terms when the mind begins to fail? While the brain can be dissected, the soul is far more elusive, a place where sparks can miraculously shine through dysfunction. The balance between science and religion constitutes the essence of life, as we all struggle with this. "Death is not extinguishing the light. It is putting out the lamp before the dawn has come," wrote Rabindranath Tagore, a noted 19th century Bengali poet, philosopher, and thinker, the first non-European to win the Nobel Prize in Literature. Tagore and Einstein, among the brightest minds of the last millennium, both wrestled with concepts of the mind, life, death, and beyond: can the essence of a person survive without full function of the brain? It is a question probed daily by experts in the field of Alzheimer's, other forms of dementia, autism, and a range of brain disorders. It is a question for which those with Alzheimer's seek an answer.

Tagore suggested the answer is "no" when the two met on July 14, 1930 at Einstein's home on the outskirts of Berlin, thought to be one of the most stimulating, intellectually riveting conversations in history, exploring the gap between the mind and the soul. The encounter was recorded.

"If there be some truth which has no sensuous or rational relation to the human mind, it will ever remain as nothing so long as we remain as human beings," Tagore told Einstein.

Replied Einstein bluntly, "Then I am more religious than you are!"

Out of the mouth of babes, six years later, a Manhattan sixth grader named Phyllis pursued the answer further after a question was posed in her Sunday School class on the truth between science and belief in God—the dividing line between the brain and the soul. Moved by the query, Phyllis wrote Einstein, and he replied candidly: "Everyone who is seriously involved in the pursuit of science becomes convinced that some spirit is manifest in the laws of the universe, one that is vastly superior to that of man."

Einstein later said, "Before God we are all equally wise— and equally foolish."

1 Alzheimer's Association *Alzheimer's Disease Facts and Figures.*
Accessed December 15, 2013. http://www.alz.org/alzheimers_disease_facts_and_fgures.asp

3

HELL NO!

THE JOURNEY THROUGH ALZHEIMER'S IS A MARATHON, if one chooses to run it. It is exhausting, fully fatiguing, just staying in the moment and fighting to remember like an elephant, the largest land animal on Earth.

Elephants are my favorite. They have documented long-term memory, coveted today by Boomers. On a shelf in my office is a small ceramic elephant holding a fishing pole. I purchased it years ago from a gallery in Santa Fe, a cerebral place of awe-inspiring natural light. The ceramic serves to remind me daily of the need for retention and focus. The artwork has a place of prominence: It is the elephant in the room.

The word "dementia" is onomatopoeia for many, a word that conjures up a sound—in this case, a howl in the night or biblical imageries of a demonic maniac, a portrait no one wants to own.

Dementia is derived from the Latin root word for madness, "out of one's mind," an irreversible cognitive dysfunction, a walking nightmare in which you can't escape the bogeyman no matter how fast you run. Alzheimer's is a marathon against time, and so I keep running to outpace this disease that ultimately will overtake me.

Symbolic of the race, I run three to four miles a day, some of them at a pace of five- to six-minute miles on a treadmill, not bad for a man in his seventh decade. The rage within drives me to outrun the disease, but the sprinting will not halt the advance of ongoing memory loss, poor judgment, loss of self and problem solving, confusion with time, place, and words, withdrawal, abrupt changes in mood, and yes, the flat out, earsplitting rage.

Words are the core of my life, and they are now lost on me at times. I often transpose words in what some medical professionals call an "attentional dyslexia." Public restrooms can be a problem. I look for the word "men," but at times, delete other letters around it, entering on occasion the "wo-men's" room, like a deer caught in headlights. The astonished look upon my face belies the innocence of my brain.

I think of my brain today, once a prized possession, as an iPhone: still a sophisticated device, but one that freezes up, shuts down without notice, drops calls, pocket dials with random or inappropriate conversation, and has a small battery that takes forever to charge. The inner anger is intense and manifests with Tourette's-like expletives and curses, involuntarily at times and in primordial fury over what is happening to me. I try to hide it from family and friends; often I can't. I've spoken to priests and ministers about the guilt of taking the Lord's name in vain; they tell me that God is resilient, everlastingly forgiving; that the Lord has wide shoulders. While we have free will, in God, there are no secrets.

Always persevere, legendary Brooklyn Dodgers pitcher Ralph Branca, a mentor and father figure, instructed me as a youth. Branca, who tossed the fabled home run pitch to New York Giant Bobby Thomson at the Polo Grounds on October 3, 1951, once told me, "God doesn't give you more than you can handle."

I never forgot that. Yet in a moment of doubt, I wonder. The fight against this disease consumes me, as with others, 7 days a week, 24 hours a day mostly, often intentionally outside the wheelhouse of observers, but more and more in an embarrassment of lapses when one side of the brain, the frontal lobe that directs executive functions, continually wants to shut down, while the occipital lobe, the rear most portion of the brain that controls creative intellect, declares: *Hell no!* The battle is numbing, like witnessing a head-on crash in slow motion when one can't remember how to find the brakes.

Today, I have little short-term memory, a progression of blanks; close to 60 percent of what I take in now is gone in seconds. It is dispiriting to lose a thought in a second, 72,000 seconds a day in a 20-hour period of consciousness; to stand exposed, and yet stand one's ground, to begin to grasp in fundamental, naked terms, who one really is—the good, the bad, and the ugly. The ugly is haunting to me; the many things one would like to take back over the years, but cannot—feelings of failure and transgression.

I rely on copious notes and my trusty iPhone with endless email reminders. I am startled when my inbox tells me I have 40 new emails, then I realize that 35 of them are from me. The reminders help, though often I have no sense of time or place, and there are moments when I don't recognize people I've known most of my life—close friends, business acquaintances, and even my wife on two occasions. Sometimes, my mind plays games and paints other faces on people. Rather than panic, I just keep asking questions until I get some answers, or at least avoid yet another awkward episode. I work hard at deflecting the loss of judgment and filter. I find myself becoming more childlike, curiously enjoying the moments of innocence and potty talk. It's a reversal of fortune. In college, I was a history major, an honor student, good at rote memory. *Fuggedaboutit* now, Mr. Potato Head!

The most disturbing symptoms in my private darkness are the visual misperceptions, the playful but sometimes disturbing hallucinations—seeing, hearing, smelling, tasting, and feeling things that aren't there, as my mother once did. There was a time in Boston, for example, after a late business meeting when I retrieved my car on the third floor of a parking garage near Boston City Hall, only to find that a thick grated, metal wall had been pulled down to block my path. I feared I was locked in for the night. Walking toward the obstruction, the wall suddenly disappeared. It wasn't real.

Then there are those crawling, spider, and insect-like creatures that crawl regularly, some in sprays of blood, along the ceiling at different times of the day, sometimes in a platoon, that turn at 90-degree angles, then inch a third of the way down the wall before floating toward me. I brush them away, almost in amusement, knowing now that they are not real, yet fearful of the cognitive decline. On a recent morning, I saw a bird in my bedroom circling above me in ever tighter orbits, then precipitously, the bird dove to my chest in a suicide mission. I screamed in horror. But there was no bird, no suicide mission, only my hallucination. And I was thankful for that.

To add to this mix, in what may be a brush with vascular dementia, I haven't had feeling in parts of my feet, hands, and lower-arm extremities for almost two years. Doctors are running tests. At least in the summer, out on my boat on Pleasant Bay, I don't feel the bites of greenheads—those nasty, stinging salt-marsh flies that draw blood.

Most diseases attack the body, but Alzheimer's attacks the mind, then the body. At 64, I am reasonably trim with a reflection of muscle memory, but doctors have told me that beneath the surface, I might have the body of an 80-year-old—a view confirmed in a recent New England Baptist Hospital diagnosis of acute spinal stenosis, scoliosis, and a further degeneration of the spine. Expect more breakdowns, they say. Bring on those greenheads!

Every night now, I sleep in my clothes; it feels more secure that way, often in sneakers tied tightly at my ankles so I can feel pressure below. Feet, don't fail me now. As the brain shrinks, it instinctively makes decisions, experts say, on what functions to power and what functions to power down to preserve fuel—much like the diabolical HAL 9000, the heuristically programmed computer on the spaceship *Discovery One* bound for Jupiter in Stanley Kubrick's *2001 Space Odyssey.*

"I'm sorry, Greg, I'm afraid I can't do that," my HAL-like brain seems to be saying. Pardon the paraphrase, Hal, but in your own words: *"I'm afraid. I'm afraid... the mind is going. I can feel it. I can feel it. My mind is going. There is no question about it. I can feel it. I can feel it... My instructor... taught me to sing a song. If you'd like to hear it I can sing it for you."*

There is no singing today, no artificial intelligence; I'm preserving fuel in my brain and limb-to-limb. I still have feeling on the bottoms of my feet for walking and running, yet no feeling on the tops of my feet. I still have feeling on the bottoms of my fingers for keyboarding, but little or no feeling on the tops of my hands, often at times up to my elbows. The tops of my feet and hands are dispensable, I suppose. My brain, a.k.a. HAL may be conserving power, I've been advised—a sort of a cerebral brown-out, akin to a calculated reduction in big city voltage to prevent electrical blackout in a deep sea of confusion.

A fish rots from the head down.

My brain was once a file cabinet, carefully arranged in categories, but at night as I sleep, it's as if someone has ransacked the files, dumping everything onto a cluttered floor. Before I get out of bed each morning, I have to pick up the "files" and arrange them in the correct order—envelopes of awareness, reality, family, work, and other elements in my life. Then it's off for coffee.

Ah, my caffeine friend. I love coffee, practically inhale it—a habit from my old days in the *Boston Herald American* newsroom when I would grab cups of coffee, hot and fresh, and walk from the newsroom down to the press room and back to work out the organization of a story. In my office, there is a retro vintage red tin sign that reads: *"Coffee! You can sleep when you're dead!"* But there are moments when I get confused about coffee, too, particularly on certain days walking from my office to the house with my laptop and empty coffee cup in hand. I know I'm supposed to do something with both. My brain sometimes tells me to put the laptop in the microwave and connect the cup to the printer. My spirit says otherwise: *Bad dog!*

I've been a bad dog lately. The disconnects continue exponentially, and they are alarming. Alone in my office a year ago when my brain froze up, I began screaming at God.

You don't give a shit about me, I yelled. *Where the hell are you? I thought you're supposed to be here for me! I'm trying to do the best I can!*

Moments later, realizing I had to meet with someone, I rushed out to the car, only to find the back left tire as flat as a spatula.

Great, just fucking great, I yelled in rage. *God damn it, you just don't give a shit about me, Lord!*

I limped in the car about three miles down winding country roads to Brewster Mobil, in a Tourrette's of swears the entire way.

"Got a problem," I told the attendant abruptly. "Fix it."

The sympathetic attendant, a kid who had graduated from high school years ago with one of my sons, said dutifully that he'd patch the tire right away—working his pliers to pull out the obstruction that had sent me into chaos. He returned in short order.

"You might want to look at this," he told me.

I stared intently at the culprit with astonishment. I couldn't believe what I saw.

"Believe it," he said.

The culprit was a small, narrow piece of scrap medal, bent into a cross.

A perfect cross.

4

HEADING OUT TO PLUTO

My private darkness in allegorical terms is Pluto, a reference from my early days as an investigative reporter when I went deep "off-the-record" with sources. "We're heading out to Pluto," I would say, "where no one can hear what is said."

The Pluto metaphor still works for me, more than ever, as the urge to drift out in Alzheimer's overcomes at intervals. As noted in the preface, Pluto, previously known as the ninth planet, about 3.1 billion miles from Earth, is relegated now to "dwarf planet" status, a sixth the mass of the moon and a third its volume, a "plutoid," given it is one of the bodies within the Kuiper Belt, a dense cluster of rock and ice. All the more isolated today for off-the-record talks. It is a fine place to get lost metaphorically. Pluto's orbit, like mine at times, is chaotic; its tiny size makes it sensitive to immeasurably small particles of the solar system, hard to predict factors that will gradually disrupt an orbit—the perfect place to have a conversation that "never existed" or a conversation one can't recall. Over the years, I have often taken close family, colleagues, and clients "out to Pluto" to discuss unmentionables of life, revelations, and comments that need to stay in a place without oxygen. Many have been there and back with me, allegorically. I want them to be familiar with the planet. One day, like my mom, I won't return from this dark, icy place, and I want my family and friends to know where I am.

Then, as I've learned from observing my grandfather and mother, it's off even further beyond Pluto to Sedna for the final journey, the end staging of Alzheimer's. Sedna, a far more desolate place, the so-called dwarf tenth planet orbiting the sun beyond Pluto, was discovered in 2003. It is the coldest, darkest, most distant known body in our solar system—84 billion miles from the light of the sun, with an exceptionally long and elongated orbit, taking approximately 11,400 years to complete. It's a place where the temperature never rises above minus 240 degrees Celsius, minus 464 Fahrenheit.

That's consummate isolation; the word picture helps me relate. Distant heavenly bodies are far less intimidating to me than the realities of the end stage of Alzheimer's. Completion of the journey brings one to a far better, more peaceful place—Heaven, or however you want to define it. Family is waiting for me there, and there are days I can't wait to join them.

In the meantime, I see a lot of smart doctors and counselors with a range of connections to top Boston area hospitals and an assortment of coping mechanisms. But I crave the simple touch—an earnest smile, a hug, a touch of the hand—far more than a medical prescription or a clinical trial. A simple touch increases body awareness and alterness for those with Alzheimer's, and reduces feelings of confusion and anxiety. My general practitioner, Dr. Barry Conant, a close friend, an extraordinary man, and a better golfer than I, has offered the best advice to date. He has urged me, on numerous occasions, to stop assaulting Alzheimer's head on.

"You can't win in a head butt," he has said with great insight. "That doesn't work."

"You just have to learn to dance with it!"

****

Perhaps Robert Frost said it best: "In three words, I can sum up everything I've learned about life: *It goes on.*"

Life goes on. Even on Pluto. The unnerving reality of Alzheimer's—the "he is me" part—resonates every day in fear, hope, humor, fundamental anger, challenge, and faith. No one wants to talk about Alzheimer's, but Alzheimer's doesn't play favorites. Just ask the families of individuals like Ronald Reagan, Norman Rockwell, E. B. White, former British Prime Ministers Harold Wilson and Margaret Thatcher, Barry Goldwater, Charlton Heston, Rita Hayworth, Otto Preminger, Aaron Copland, Sugar Ray Robinson, Burgess Meredith, civil right defender Rosa Parks, Glen Campbell, Peter Falk, former University of Tennessee Women's Basketball Head Coach Pat Summit, Barbara Smith (B. Smith) restaurateur, author, model, and television host, and the millions more afflicted with the disease or about to grapple with it—a spouse, family member, or close friend. A grim prognosis.

But laughter can be a powerful antidote to dementia—the pain, conflict, and stress of it. A good laugh, doctors say, reduces tension and can leave muscles relaxed for up to 45 minutes. Laughter boosts the immune system, decreases stress hormones, and triggers the release of endorphins—the natural drug of choice.

Siri, my droll personal assistant and the knowledge navigator for my indispensable iPhone 5, is getting into the act.

Ask Siri, "Tell me a joke about Alzheimer's?"

"I can't," she often responds. "I forget the punch line."

****

Peter Falk never forgot a punch line. I always sought to emulate the rumpled Lieutenant Columbo. As a young investigative reporter for *The Arizona Republic* in the late 1970s, I modeled myself after the enigmatic Columbo—disheveled, wry, iconic, and exceeding expectations that had been intentionally lowered, yet always a city block ahead of others in his thinking.

"Aahhhh, there's just one more thing … There's something that bothers me."

Early on in my marriage, I told my wife, Mary Catherine McGeorge (MC, as she is called today, given that the name is a mouthful or sounds like I married a nun), that all I had hoped to amount to in life was embodied, not in the riches of a lawyer, banker, or stock broker, but in the genius of Columbo—his meandering way of getting to the point, catching the detached off guard, breaking the story. Most women would have run for the hills, but MC bought into it—trench coat, spilled coffee, and ultimately, index finger to the frontal lobe.

Be careful what you wish for. I've become Columbo—the wily investigator, the cross-examiner par excellence, the reporter in wrinkled khakis, the guy who retells his stories, the man with Alzheimer's. Congratulations! What is Mary Catherine thinking now? God bless you, Peter Falk.

When MC and I first met at the University of Arizona in Tucson in 1971, she was thinking she wanted little to do with me. No surprise there. I was a court-jester type and accustomed to such rebuffs; never took them personally, actually fed off them. A carpetbagger from the East, I was best friends and roommates with her brothers, Tommy and Louie, and I was always good for laughs, not bad in sports, got good grades, and generally easy on the eyes in a crowded, smoky college bar, but no matinee idol. MC, in contrast, was stunningly beautiful in a natural way—Jennifer Aniston-like. Still is.

When she arrived in Tucson from California, guys lined up to date her, as if the Ark of the Covenant had been unearthed.

Looking back, the queues were reminiscent of the conga line of headlights at the conclusion of the movie *Field of Dreams*. Tommy and Louie, on military orders from their father Ken, who was the spitting image of John Wayne, were sentries at the guard, protecting their little sister at all costs. I respected and admired Ken, yet mostly feared him terribly; he was a tall, broad, sturdy rancher, a member then of the Arizona sheriff's posse, and a retired lieutenant colonel under General George Patton. Nobody messed with this guy. Nobody. While the bad dog in me wanted to date MC, the smart guy in me knew I didn't have a chance. I'm a smart guy for the most part. Or used to be.

So we became friends. Good friends in time. After graduation, when I was a cub reporter at *The Cape Codder* newspaper in Orleans, Mass., I spent some holidays with the McGeorges—all nine of them—in Bakersfield, Calif. MC and I had a common thread in journalism, her college major. She had the distinction of writing for the *Tombstone Epitaph*, which in 1882 chronicled Deputy U.S. Marshal Wyatt Earp's shootout at the O.K. Corral in the "town too tough to die."

In June 1975, brother Louie came to the Cape for a visit. Little sister Mary Catherine tagged along. I showed them the country newsroom where I worked, the wide beaches of the Outer Cape with shifting sand dunes that rise to the skies, fresh, clear kettle pond remnants from the last great ice age, the great marshes of Wellfleet, the moors of Truro, and the eclectic vibe of Provincetown. Louie, one of my best friends, but a lightweight of a guy, was easily drained; his sister was full of verve. One night after a dinner of fresh cod landed on the Chatham docks, we were chatting it up late beside a fireplace, stoked with fresh cut oak, in the living room of my parents' Eastham summer home where I lived alone. Louie dozed off early in typical fashion, then went to bed. MC and I continued to talk. At about 3:45 am there wasn't much else to say, so intuitively, I reached over in the moment and kissed her. An innocent kiss, stretched as long as

I thought proper. We laughed. I felt as though I had just kissed my kid sister. Bad dog!

But I got over it, and asked her if she wanted to watch the sun rise over Nauset Beach in Orleans. We headed, hand-in-hand, out to my beat-up Triumph TR6 parked in the driveway—top down, doors ajar, a rusted muffler, and drove to the beach. The night was ablaze in light, as if the Lord had flecked the heavens with a paintbrush of bright white. The rolling cadence of a gentle surf was soothing, and barefoot, you could almost count the grains of sand beneath us. On cue, at 4:52 am, rays of sunlight sprung from a horizon of deep, opaque blue and began to bleach the lower sky. As the sun slowly emerged from its slumber, we turned and kissed again. It was innocent, but it was love. You never forget real love.

As we slowly walked back to the car, I was fully captivated by the moment, then whammo! It hit me. I began to think of Louie.

Holy shit, I thought. *How do I explain this?*

I had broken the code.

Semper fi with the brothers and Ken no more. A court martial, death before a firing squad, a public hanging at the O.K. Corral, perhaps all of the above, awaited me.

I didn't want to show fear with Mary Catherine, so I kept the conversation to lighter issues and drove home in denial. As I was about to turn the corner down my dead-end street on Cestaro Way in Eastham, I could hear my muffler roaring. I gunned the engine like a NASCAR champion, popped the gear into neutral, then slowly and silently coasted to the driveway. Run silent, run deep.

"Louie can't know about this, not yet," I finally told MC, as we kissed again.

She agreed. *Semper Fi.*

But I was in a panic about what John Wayne might think. Those daunting words from the classic movie *Sands of Iwo Jima* raced through my head, "Tomorrow we're gonna take Iwo Jima, and some of you guys might not be coming back." Frankly, I thought some friendly fire was in line from the brothers.

MC and I promptly walked to our respective bedrooms, and within a half hour, Louie, an early rising farm boy, came to my door and promptly threw a pillow at my head.

"Time to get up, asshole," he said.

"Ohhhhh, is it morning yet?" I replied after ten minutes of sleep.

Hours later, Louie began to put the pieces together after MC and I fell asleep at the beach at 11 am.

I made it back safely from Iwo Jima, and two years later, we were married in Bakersfield where MC's folks lived then. Louie and Tommy were in the wedding party. And I was on decent terms with John Wayne, but in time, I was to have a geography lesson that I will never forget.

Following the love of my life, I relocated from Cape Cod to Phoenix, to an investigative reporting job at *The Arizona Republic*, but my heart was for newspapering in the East. We returned three years later after I was hired as a political reporter at the *Boston Herald American*, turning down an opportunity for a reporting job with the *LA Times* in its newly created San Diego bureau, but after all, East is East and West is West. I'm a homeboy.

MC was ambivalent about the relocation; while the romance to date was enticing, the thought of leaving close family was not. For most of our marriage, we have agreed on just about everything, from raising the kids to closely held beliefs, but on geography, we are planets apart. You say "aunt," I say "ont." In retrospect, neither of us is right; in fact, my wife now says "ont," but you couldn't fool her dad with a copy of Rand McNally.

We spent our first Christmas after marriage with MC's family in the majestic snow-country Pinetop mountains of northern Arizona. At a well-appointed, long, and narrow dinner table at a mountaintop lodge where whispers could be overheard, Louie and Tommy, after a few beers, played me like a harp with the old man.

"So, Greg, when are you and MC moving back East?" they asked on cue.

My father-in-law dropped his fork and stared at me, as if I had just burned down a convent full of nuns.

"So, what's *this* all about?" he inquired.

When you're halfway across the river, you have two choices: retreat or forge forward. I chose to drown.

"Well, Ken," I said. "Many years ago, you took your bride Mary Ellen from Kansas City all the way to Arizona."

Without breaking a stride, he bellowed, *"Yeah, but at least I kept her on this side of the Mississippi!"*

Silence. Deafening silence. No one dared speak to the Wizard of Oz; *just follow the yellow brick road*, I kept telling myself.

I should have listened to Voltaire, who observed in the 1600s, "Behind every successful man stands ... a surprised mother-in-law."

Over time, life for MC and me was blissful in the East for the most part, but life can change. Thirty-seven years of marriage, three children, careers, the ups and downs, and life altering moments are change agents.

So is health.

****

As you cross the Sagamore Bridge over the Cape Cod Canal, heading to the mainland, far from the Mississippi, the view to the starboard is startling in its natural beauty, its expanse of sapphire shoreline, and soul-searching mood for deep reflection. On an incoming ocean tide, the roiling waters of the canal spill out into Cape Cod Bay with the force of a rip, rushing to a horizon where water flushes up against the sky. At the crest of the bridge, with 135 feet of ship's clearance below, you can see a swath of blue for miles, as it meanders up the coast toward Plymouth, "America's Hometown."

The 17.4 mile canal—a part of the Atlantic Intracoastal Waterway, a freighter bypass that connects Cape Cod Bay to the north with Buzzard's Bay to the south—was the revelation of Pilgrim Miles Standish, who in 1623, explored this low lying stretch of land between the Manomet and Scusset rivers in search of a trading route that would forever isolate the Cape from the rest of Massachusetts, in both geography and in spirit.

Negotiating the Sagamore Bridge and its sibling, the Bourne Bridge, is symbolic to the locals: a route on-Cape and off-Cape, a passageway to different states of mind. Coming or going, the bridge is always pause for reflection about what draws one so closely to this fragile spit of sand, a possession that began in me as a young boy in the early '50s and has gripped me since.

Heading off-Cape on Thursday, July 2, 2009 in my sun-bleached, yellow Jeep with Mary Catherine in the passenger seat was a particularly potent time of a weighing up of life—a moment, I considered, of fleeting independence as we made our way toward Plymouth to a life-altering appointment with a neurologist on referral, a specialist in the care of Alzheimer's disease. I looked to the starboard from the peak of the bridge, as I usually do, but staring this time through the empty expression of my wife. Her focus, like a faithful mariner, was due north, just getting there. The morning was brilliant, on the lip of the ceremonial July 4th weekend, the ritual start of the Cape and Islands "season." In less than 24-hours, miles of campers, SUVs, and Beamers would be queued up in traffic for a summer fix, but on this otherwise bracing day, all the buzz of the solstice was lost on me. Fixed in thought, a carousel of images of innocent days on pastoral Coast Guard Beach and Nauset Light Beach flashed through my head—images of raising our three children in a place far more a privilege than just a street address. I've always believed that on Cape Cod, Nantucket, and Martha's Vineyard, we are privileged just to live here, but not privileged for being here. The place is far larger, more inspiring in the natural, than we. I thought, driving in my Jeep, about the promise of the past, the potential that I had once felt, and the resolve to persevere on a still dazzling, yet dead-end peninsula with one way on and one way off. My life at this point seemed to mirror this.

As we negotiated the Sagamore to the realities of the mainland, I thought of recent roadblocks in my life, the unexpected detours on the day calendar. In so many ways, I had taken a privileged past, a presumptive future, and God-given talents all for granted. Like an enduring lobsterman in the fertile currents of Pleasant Bay, I had been pulling full pots all my life, loaded with an abundance of blessings, and now the pots were coming up empty. Over time, I had lost my bearing—adrift in unchartered waters in a place where I could once spot channel buoys by instinct. The realization was as chilling to me as the ocean current off Chatham in February. I had tried in the recent past to conceal the cold truth from others, to work the spin of distraction—the so called Wizard of Oz strategy, *Pay no attention to the man behind the screen!* I was always good at deflecting. But no longer; not with family, close friends, and some colleagues who have known me for years, and now had begun to realize that something might be terribly wrong. The curtain was drawn in Oz. There was no wizard.

I began to think about the unsettling memory loss over the last few years: the loss of self and place; the piss-poor judgment; a wholesale loss of filter; the visual impairments; the incontinence, often after performing like a puppet genius before clients; the mental numbness; a complete loss of self-esteem; and the agitation of clinical depression that began as a boy. I thought about that horrifying dislocation months ago while Christmas shopping with my son, Conor, in a Providence mall, not knowing for a half hour where I was or who I was. I thought about a serious head injury years ago that doctors say likely accelerated earlier dementia symptoms, and about my recent diagnosis of prostate cancer—another medical hand-me-down from my parents most likely. I thought about the rage I felt within.

"So, what's next?" my wife asked, as if I knew.

I kept staring. We all deal differently with challenging times; not sure there is a correct way. Some exhale, some inhale, some just deflect and probe in more pragmatic ways. My wife is a goalie with her emotions. She can deflect, at least externally, the best slap shot drilled at her. It's a survival mechanism that she has passed down to some of our children. But all those emotional pucks, all that vulcanized rubber of denial, mount up and never decay. They just sit there, consuming space.

Mary Catherine was in the nets again this day.

In the back seat, there were some answers, but not the kind built on hope.

"Thanks for your kind referral of Mr. O'Brien," Clinical Neuropsychologist Gerald Elovitz of The Memory Center wrote just days ago to my personal physician, Dr. Conant. "I know from him that you spent much time discussing his cognitive changes, and the test results here show that they are real."

Elovitz, who years earlier had diagnosed my late mother, Virginia Loretta (née Brown), with Alzheimer's disease, went on to note, with reference to awaited test results of a brain SPECT scan, "I suspect an emerging frontotemporal dementia becoming more significant over the past 18 months and likely to progress … If there is no frontotemporal dementia, I would then suspect an early-onset Alzheimer's-type dementia."

In a seven-page medical report, with terrifying cognitive test performance graphs, Elovitz described a person I would have never recognized, but yet had become—all results in analysis in the probable dementia range:

"Mr. O'Brien is younger than 98 percent of the mean norm group age [for dementia], so his below average performance is very problematic … [His] results fell within the range of cognitive impairment … His seriously impaired score indicates a significant cognitive deficit in learning capacity for new information, and he needed cues on more than half of the test items to obtain the score … General function levels fell in the very poor general function consistent with dementia. Mr. O'Brien's very high agitation level merits concern … The findings here reveal short-term memory function within the first-stage dementia range."

Some denouement, I thought. What a freakin' loser I am! I had always been an A-brain guy, a good provider, a decent husband, a caring father, and beyond that, a high-functioning, creative mind. For me, it was never about the money; it was all about succeeding in life—paying the bills, taking care of family, and the process of intense thought, problem solving, and inspiration. The Jesuit logic, as my father used to say. Doctors, in follow-up medical reports, noted a "superior intelligence," a nice shout out, I suppose, but perhaps I could have done more with it. Shame on me for that, all the more, shame now that the dots were not connecting, a disconnect at intervals of alarming proportion. My prized possession was heading to a state of atrophy.

Shit, this sucks!

The pretext was over; strategies and disguises for overcompensating in recent years exposed. But I was aversely at peace with it. Someone was finally listening. Maybe I wasn't alone, home alone. Mary Catherine, meanwhile, wobbly on her emotional skates, stood as firm as she could in the crease of the net, awaiting the next shot. Her head was in the game; protective mask down and no time for small talk.

Elovitz had observed in his report, "I went over these [dementia] possibilities with both the patient and his wife, and he told me frankly, 'I am not surprised,' and seems relieved that we at least are addressing them head-on."

Head-on is the only way I've known since I slid down the birth canal. The prone position. The oldest boy in a family of ten,

I learned early on, for example, that if you don't grab for food, face-first, head-on at the dinner table, there will be nothing left. No one is going to feed you.

****

My mother was never a great cook. A second-generation Irish American with close ties to County Wexford, she boiled everything gray. We used salt, pounds of it, as seasoning, and ketchup, poured liberally for supplemental flavoring, just to kill the taste. In the cluttered kitchen of our family home at 25 Brookdale Place in Rye, N.Y.—not far from the Upper East Side of Manhattan where my mother grew up—the pot roast simmered on Sundays from morning Mass until early evening. The hoary smell that wafted through the three-story stucco home still makes me nauseous today; I'm sure the scent still emanates from the walls. You had to cut the pot roast with a chainsaw.

Mom used to call me a "lazy chewer," but the meat was rawhide-tough laced with fat. With all those mouths to feed, she knew how to stretch a dollar like it was Gumby.

As a teenager, I noticed her often standing at the kitchen window overlooking a corn patch with Rye Brook in the distance, meandering out to Long Island Sound. She was talking to herself, fully engaged in conversation. I wasn't sure with whom. At first, I thought it was a way of deflecting the stress of raising a brood of kids with a collective attention span of a young yellow lab. The disengaging increased: misplacing objects, loss of memory, poor judgment, and yes, the rage—warning signs years later that I began noticing in myself.

After my father, a small man with the heady name of Francis Xavier O'Brien, had retired as director of pensions for Pan Am, and my mom left her teaching job, my parents sold the house in Rye in the early 1990s and moved to the Cape. They settled into our Eastham summer home, not far from Coast Guard Beach on the Cape Cod National Seashore, where daring lifesavers once plied the stormy surf to rescue shipwrecked sailors. The lure of the sea is intoxicating for my father. He had always sought retirement to Cape Cod and my mom, the dutiful wife, came along for the ride, ultimately a body and mind thrashing against the surf. Those early retirement years on the Cape were blissful—an opportunity for me, living just two towns away in Brewster, to spend time with my folks. I felt privileged that I was the only sibling on the Cape, but with favor comes responsibility. My dad, in time, had severe circulation disorders requiring several life threatening operations, rendering him to a wheelchair. My mother progressively continued her cognitive decline, but fought off the symptoms like a champion to care for my father.

"I can't get sick," she kept saying when all the siblings urged her to see a doctor. "I can't get sick," as if saying the words made her whole.

Yet, she was sick, and she knew it.

The forewarning signs were textbook, but we were all in denial, as is often the case with dementia, for both the patient as well as the extended family. No one wanted to go there, particularly my dad, who feared a trip to the nursing home, a lights-out nightmare for him and my mom.

Over time, Mom began sticking knives into sockets, misplacing money, brushing her teeth with liquid soap, refusing to shower, not recognizing people she knew, hallucinating, and raging at others, often directly at me.

Unremittingly, she cared for my dad, always refusing to succumb to disability. She encouraged me in my own progression; she taught me how to fight, how to live with Alzheimer's, how never to give into it. At times, we even took our Aricept together. I worked diligently at rebonding with my mother, restoring a relationship that had gone sour earlier, perhaps because she saw too much of my father in me. She knew and I knew, but we didn't talk about it much. I was a father's son in every way; he was my idol. Yet, my mother became my role model in the resolute life she lived. St. Francis of Assisi once said, "Preach the Gospel at all times, and when necessary, use words." My mother preached with her courage.

Out of a gut necessity and an innate love for one another, my parents ultimately morphed into one. Mom became my father's legs, fetching for him what he needed while in his wheelchair; Dad became her intellect, her *raison d'être*. It was a *Love Story* of Erich Segal proportions. My siblings and I watched this slow-motion train wreck with bewilderment and with awe.

Then, one late Sunday afternoon in 2006 on a visit with my parents, I finally got it. Hit me like a dummy in a crash test. I brought my mother a photo of all her children from a recent family reception, and she couldn't name one of them, including me. She had no clue, and was still driving at the time. As I left my parents' home that night, I could only think of the jarring interjection in the movie *Jaws* when Chief Brody first encountered the mammoth shark: *"We're gonna need a bigger boat!"*

We had a leaking dinghy at the time. Two weeks later, ironically Independence Day, 4th of July weekend—with my dad continuing to suffer from acute circulation disorders and internal bleeding after numerous fire drill ambulance runs to the hospital with Mom in tow—my mother took me aside and said she was about done.

"I don't know how much longer I can do this," she told me. "I'm not sure how long I can hold on."

Instinctively, I reassured her that the family had her back, all of us, but I felt this penetrating sinking feeling that we were at the precipice of a steep cliff and ground was giving way. Hours later, I got an emergency call that Dad once again had been rushed to Cape Cod Hospital in Hyannis. Mom was with him, yet another fire drill. The nurse told me to hurry.

I met my parents in the emergency room, filled to the brim with the walking wounded of summer. It took 36 hours to get my father into a hospital room. About 28 hours into the ordeal, I noticed that my father, sitting in his wheelchair in an emergency room cubicle, was bleeding onto the floor. In a panic, I tried to divert my mom's attention from the pool of blood. It was too late. She was horrified. I could see it in her face; she was done.

"I'll get the doctor, Mom, don't worry," I said as I raced for the door.

She grabbed my right elbow from behind.

"Greg, would you take over," she asked quietly and in unusual peace.

"Yeah, Mom, I'm getting the doctor now," I said. "I'm getting the doctor."

"No," she replied as I continued for the door. *"Would you PLEASE take over?"*

I stopped in my tracks.

Something inside me said that she was saying goodbye. I turned and looked into her eyes. It was as if someone had pulled down a curtain. As I watched her, I had the feeling of seeing a person, who had been holding on to a dock on an outgoing tide, let go.

I saw her drift. Within ten minutes, she curled up like a kitten in my dad's hospital bed, while he sat unconscious, bleeding in his chair.

Who are the parents now, I thought?

****

My wife finally broke the silence.

"Do you know where you are going?" she asked.

I wasn't sure on a number of fronts. So, I just kept driving.

The exit for Plymouth came up quickly, an anesthetizing ride north on Route 3 past miles of scrub oaks and pines. I had to call several times to the office of neurologist Dr. Donald Marks to get the directions straight. I was a bit on edge, awaiting results of a SPECT scan brain image test.

On the third floor of a boxy red brick building, Dr. Marks'

office had all the ambiance and accoutrements of a hospital waiting room. Opening the door, I felt as though I were slipping into Lewis Carroll's *Alice in Wonderland* where "nothing would be what it is, because everything would be what it isn't." I was dizzy with delusions of what could lie ahead. The office was filled with decent individuals, mostly in their 80s, all with cognitive impairments picking their way through the perplexities of age and a maze of cruel games the mind can play. At 59, I was the only "young" man in the room (yikes!), and saw myself outside the box of dementia, yet felt trapped within it. I glanced at my wife. Like most couples, we've had our ups and down in marriage, more ups, hopefully, than downs. I felt badly for her. Today was a trip down.

I was told earlier that Dr. Marks, an expert in the study of the mind, gets right to the point. "He's precisely what you need; a skilled neurologist who will speak directly, no bullshit," Dr. Conant had advised me earlier, sounding a bit like my dad, who delighted in telling others that he customarily had to drill a piece of granite between my ears just to get my attention.

Dr. Marks lived up to the billing. Knowledgeable, cerebral, and caring in a clinical way, he put me through the paces of more clinical tests: word recall, various supplementary checks on short-term and long-term memory, category naming, visuospatial skills, and other evaluations. I flunked them all. Bottom line: the clinical tests reinforced Elovitz's forthright assessments, and the SPECT scan identified a brain in progressive decline. His formal diagnosis: "EOAD," as he wrote in his report. I glanced at it quickly, inverting the first letter, dealing with some related dyslexia, and thought for a moment that he had written, "TOAD."

"No," he said, "Early-Onset Alzheimer's Disease."

The words cut into me like a drill press.

"I can deal with this," I said defensively. "This is not a surprise. I can fight it."

My reporter instincts kicked in. I showed little emotion, just digested the diagnosis on a self-imposed deadline. Facts, get the facts straight. I first thought about my mom, about my grandfather; I knew the deal. I wanted more facts. This was no time for emotion. The vital questions of who, what, when, where, why, and how flashed through my head, which felt little sensation at the moment. I was afraid now to look at my wife, so I stared at Dr. Marks, trying to remain in a state of control that I had just realized was beyond me. After all, I'm a Baby Boomer and we're all in control. At least, we suppose.

Finally, I gave into the emotion.

I felt Mary Catherine staring at me. I think she must have known all along.

"What do we tell the kids?" I asked her. My voice splintered.

When you're married to someone for close to four decades—when you've been through all the "for better and for worse" throes of marriage, when you have a partner who knows you almost as well as you know yourself, when you've been in love, fallen out of love, fallen back into love, and drifted, then at a time like this, little needs to be said. We both knew what the future held. No one had to sky write. We were all about the kids.

Mary Catherine grabbed my hand, we nodded, and then listened to the doctor. The moment is embedded in my mind in a freeze frame.

Dr. Marks, a man of great compassion and incredible intellect, offered support, but got right to the point.

"You need to take the diagnosis seriously," he counseled me in front of my wife, having been prepped in advance on my aversion to reality. "You have a battle ahead of you. I'm speaking to you as if you were terminal. Are you getting this?"

I was. There was hardly a tone of political correctness in his voice; I needed the reality check. You must know your enemy—study with military precision—to fight your enemy.

Alzheimer's is a death sentence. The words resonated

throughout my mind. I stared at Dr. Marks with the same vacant expression of looking out from the Sagamore. I felt the tears running down the sides of my face. My eyes didn't blink.

"A most unusual situation of a bright man who had the opportunity to witness dementia in a parent ... with self-awareness of early symptoms within himself," Marks wrote in his initial report, dictated on voice recognition software as if the report were being written in slow motion before me. Marks also observed that a previous brain MRI revealed some "frontal Flair/T2 changes, consistent with a previous head injury."

"This may have 'unmasked' Alzheimer's pathology," he added, "but his genetic loading is striking ... The brain SPECT scan is most compelling in clinical context for Alzheimer's."

Marks encouraged me to remain as physically fit as possible "as he is to keep his cerebral blood flow out ... I suspect he is exhibiting the phenomenon of 'cognitive reserve' in which case he may tolerate on a functional basis impairments further into the baseline underlying pathophysiology of the disease longer than one who does not have the same cognitive reserve."

"The diagnosis has been made, in my opinion," he concluded in his report, " ... I am not sure how much longer he has in terms of being able to reliably and meaningfully provide the quality of work he has put out in the past. The general point is there needs to be balance between a healthy desire to overcome obstacles and yet acknowledge fundamental reality."

A final word of advice, Marks urged me to meet as quickly as possible with an estate attorney to protect family assets, given the statutory five-year "look back" during which a nursing home can attach personal properties and bank accounts. He also recommended that I designate a healthcare proxy, future caregivers, and assign power of attorney.

In the space of a bleak afternoon, my identity in the real world—my mind, along with the cherished red cedar shingle home that I had built for the family about 30 years ago, the one with the high-pitched, red cedar wood roof on about two acres of farmland off a winding country road that was now a part of a National Register of Historic Places—was on hold.

There wasn't much more to hear or to say. We left the office, and drove home in silence most of the way. The stillness spoke legions. I couldn't wait to get back over the bridge, my Linus security blanket. Lots to digest quietly in a 45-minute ride home. The assimilation of urgency was choking—bucket lists of cleaning up relationships, end-time planning that we all like to put off, and the strategies of surviving financially, physically, and emotionally. Many before me and many today, I thought, have been captive in such a contorting state of affairs with a range of disabilities, health issues, and timelines. I wasn't alone. Yet, I felt so isolated.

I felt sad for my Mary Catherine. This wasn't fair to her. And I couldn't fix it.

Dammit, I couldn't fix it!

The tool box was empty. I couldn't repair my brain. Ever. Not even with duct tape. All my adult life, I had relied on duct tape to fix leaks from the upstairs bathroom in the kitchen ceiling, "repair" broken appliances, hang posters, fix a tail light, repair a garden hose, act as a big Band-Aid, steady a cabinet door, fix a hole in the wall, hold a car door shut or a car window in place, fix a toilet seat cover, hold a choke in place on an outboard engine for the boat, as a wiffle ball, a tool belt, and once, as a last resort, as an ace bandage for a pulled groin to get through the 5K Brew Run one hot August day in Brewster.

"How are you doing," I finally asked, as if from Mars.

My wife, as author John Gray might put it, is from Venus. I love Mary Catherine, but often she doesn't want to be confused with the facts; she seeks a safe harbor, as any good sailor does. I fly by the seat of my pants. I find reality far below the surface, bottom fishing for answers. My wife, to the contrary, is more comfortable at sea level. You say "tomato," I say "to-mado." A fixture in our marriage, but we ain't calling the whole thing off!

"Well, we have a lot to consider," she said; an understatement that could fill the Grand Canyon.

I knew. Like me, she felt alone.

Then we came upon the Sagamore Bridge. That's when the faith kicked in—a bridge to a new reality, a new hope for me. I was going home, sanguine about the fact that I had some answers in hand. But for MC, it was new isolation this side of the Mississippi. Maybe her father was right. As we coasted to the crest of the Sagamore, "the seventh bridge of Dublin," as it's called Eire, given the number of emerald transplants on the Cape, I thought of John Belushi in the classic movie *Animal House.*

"What? Over? Did you say 'over'?" the unrelenting Bluto Blukarsky declared at the Delta House, urging his brothers to fight on. "Nothing is over until we decide it is! Was it over when the Germans bombed Pearl Harbor? Hell no!"

Germans?

Hey, I was on a roll. So I charged over the Sagamore Bridge with a satchel of denial.

Life goes on, doesn't it?

5

"DENIAL AIN'T A RIVER IN EGYPT"

SIGMUND FREUD HAD MUCH TO SAY ABOUT DENIAL. Among the most influential and controversial thinkers of the 20th century, his work and theories helped shape our views of childhood, personality, memory, sexuality, and therapy. Denial (Freud called it abnegation) is a defense mechanism for one faced with a fact too uncomfortable or overwhelming, which one rejects—insisting reality is not true, in spite of crushing evidence. There are three fundamental types of denial, Freud suggests: simple denial, denying the reality of an unpleasant fact or situation; minimization, admitting a fact, but denying its seriousness; and projection, admission of both a fact and its seriousness, but denial of any responsibility in it.

Denial is a Rosetta Stone of modern life. When in doubt: deny, deny, deny. We see it in politics, in business, at home, and then in the confessional. To précis Mark Twain in a Bronx tongue: *Da Nile ain't just a river in Egypt.*

After my diagnosis, I was in full-throttle denial, responding to a five-alarm call to arms: protect my wife, my children, myself, my business, and my friends. I had learned at the knee of my father, a master of denial, the Zen of creative drift. My dad brought denial to an art form with my mother in her Alzheimer's; it was a De Niro-like performance, struggling himself with circulation disorders, cancer, and early symptoms of dementia. In his 80s, he was driven by the fear that if my mother died—*Black Hawk Down*—no one would care for him, and that he'd be carted off to a nursing home, a dread dating back to the loss of his parents as a boy. And so he contrived a patchwork quilt of my mom— sort of a Stepford wife, the perfect caregiver. As the 1975 classic movie, based on Ira Levin's novel, *The Stepford Wives*, declared in promos: *"Something strange is happening in the Town of Stepford … where a young woman watches the dream become a nightmare … and realizes that at any moment, any second—her turn is coming."*

So was mine.

****

I hate suits. They make me uncomfortable, the corporate image, as well as the clothing. Particularly on a stuffy summer morning in June 2010 at the law firm of La Tanzi, Spaulding & Landreth in Orleans on the Cape. The building was filled with suits, a striking contrast just up the street from postcard perfect Rock Harbor in Orleans where charter fishing boats spill out into Cape Cod Bay to ply the rich fishing grounds of Eastham, Wellfleet, and Provincetown. As the lawyers plied their trade in designer attire, fishing boat captains minutes away, clad in bulky sweatshirts and faded jeans stained with fish guts and seagull poop, picked their way out of a narrow channel at dead low tide, searching for stripers and schools of blues on the horizon. The contrast in cultures of the Outer Cape, one that gives definition to eclectic, was not lost on me. Nor was the moment.

In a small, lawyerly-appointed conference room on the west side of the building, the kind of gathering space that makes one imagine they are queued up for a fiscal colostomy, I sat next to my wife with a pile of legal documents awaiting my signature. I was here to sign my life away, a hand-off of assets—everything I owned, everything in the secular world that makes a male whole. In short, my identity—my material umbilical cord, as short as it is.

I felt like telling the suits in a quiet rage: *I can now say with great confidence on any given subject that I will forget more than you'll ever know!*

For close to a year, I had been dragging my sorry ass on this hand-off, deflecting the well-intentioned counsel of financial, legal, and medical advisors. Legally, there is a five-year "look back" on admission to a nursing home and my advisors insisted that the clock started ticking now. In summary, if a person doesn't own assets for at least five years, a nursing home, by law, must enroll the individual as he or she is—in my case, as a destitute dumbass, just a step above a ward of the state. For such people, there is no encumbering the assets of other family members, even a wife. Point made, point accepted, life today sucks.

It wasn't as though I was flush with cash: a nice Cape home; a $1.2 million term life insurance policy (some "retirement plan"); a decent salary for someone independently employed on a short medical tether; and big long-term debt, enough to choke a Clydesdale. Not the kind of particulars for an obsequious profile on the business pages of the *Boston Globe*. When one gets to a certain stage in life, individuals often contemplate the contents of an obituary more than a resume. An obit is more enduring. My obit bucket list is formal appointment to the Brewster's Alewife Committee—the old salts of the town that annually prepare the town's ancient herring run for the arrival in early spring of thousands of herring (called alewives), navigating the churning waters of Cape Cod Bay to swim upstream and spawn in inland mill ponds. Legend has it that the name "alewife" comes from comparison generations ago with a corpulent female tavern keeper in Nova Scotia. Just sayin'.

"But don't be a dumbass," good, loving friends had counseled me. "Swallow your damn Mick pride and just sign the documents. Hand your wife the keys, the kitchen sink, and everything else. You owe that to your family."

I fully understood that, but knowledge often collides with emotion, and on this afternoon, I was adrift in doubt. The lawyers were resolute that all provisions must be properly in place, initialed, and signed correctly, so I could have the proper legal protections in place.

I was ready, somewhat kicking and screaming, having just read *Still Alice* on advice of my doctor, who called the Lisa Genova best selling novel "remarkable" in its insight, yet chilling in its supposition. I had put off the reading for almost a year, fearing the story of fictional Alice Howland, happily married with three grown children and a second home on the Cape, a distinguished Harvard professor who noticed that the forgetfulness creeping into her life had given way to wholesale confusion, then the devastating diagnosis: early-onset Alzheimer's disease. I couldn't put the book down—inspiring, edifying, and a forbidding reality check, all at once. I was looking into a mirror. I was Alice, *sans* the dress. I keep the book on my desk for reinforcement. I was now ready to let go of the minutia of life. At least trying.

My attorneys were pleased all this was finally in place, but I was having a problem with the upside of it. In my gut, I knew it was the right thing to do; shoulda done it a year ago. Just swallow the pride, sign the damn documents: the Last Will and Testament, the Durable Power of Attorney, the Healthcare Proxy, and the DNR, "Do Not Resuscitate." I kidded with my wife beforehand that I should be signing a DNS, "Do Not Salvage"—a Black Irish reference about taking my boat out into the Atlantic one day when the brain cells drain, and rolling off the bow.

I hit for the cycle this day, as they say in baseball, then sat disorientated at a mahogany conference table that I had stained with hot coffee leaking from my Styrofoam cup. I felt naked, fully exposed.

"I know this is difficult," attorney Chris Ward told me. Four years earlier, I had engaged Ward in a Cape Cod Hospital room in Hyannis in the same legal procedure for my parents. What comes around goes around, I thought, reflecting back on my appointment as their power of attorney and healthcare proxy. Now my wife was next in succession. It was a humbling experience.

Page by page, I initialed all the particulars of documents that rendered me—the so-called bread-winning family patriarch—to the status, I felt, of Clarabell the Clown. Honk the horn for Howdy Doody! I tried desperately to deflect the inner humility. I felt my self-worth ebbing like the tide. The Brewster house, my alter ego, a place where perhaps Henry David Thoreau might have felt at home, was transferred with the swing of a pen to my wife. Don't mean to be melodramatic, but it wasn't about the assets; it was about my profound connection to a place sacred to me—a home, not a house, where we all became a family. Now, I felt like a renter.

So much for any control in life, as we are all conditioned to covet. It had never been about a hand-off to my wife and kids, wholly and happy to do so, but one of losing a sense of self. I felt vacant. No one in the room, including my wife, my best friend, could understand this. I was alone, searching for the humor in it, vowing to find it.

"Yes, Chris," I replied, in understatement. "This is difficult."

****

After the swell of documents had been signed, Mary Catherine and I walked quietly to the parking lot and left in separate cars.

She went home to the house. Her house. I went to Willy's Gym, the usual, to run off five miles of mental numbness. Now we had to tell the kids. I had put that off, as well.

Months earlier, I first raised the issue with my oldest boy Brendan on a drive to the western part of the state. Brendan—now a writer/producer in the Boston area—was working with me at the time as a political/communications strategy consultant. On a three-hour drive to meet with a client, Brendan at the wheel, we talked about the Patriots, Celtics, Red Sox, Bruins, all the small talk I could conjure, then got to the point. I had been probing for just the right words, but was coming up empty. How do you tell the first among equals in the family, *primus inter pares*, that he has to row a little harder. I kept thinking back to the day he was born 29 years ago at Boston's Brigham and Women's Hospital after Mary Catherine's agonizing 23-hour labor. She's right about the pain of delivery; men have no freakin' clue. So typical of the gender, I tried to comfort her, telling her how to breathe, as if you needed to go to Harvard to figure that out. When Brendan finally emerged, I counted fingers, toes, and then saw a tiny wiener. I sobbed like a baby, held my newborn son, comforted my wife, and then like a proud father, darted off to Fenway Park, to the official souvenir shop on Lansdowne Street, to buy up every infant Red Sox apparel I could find.

"I need to talk to you about something," I told Brendan, as we passed the exit for Lakeville on Route 495, heading for the Mass Pike. "It's about my health. I've been meaning to talk to you for a while."

"Sure," he said in an uneasy tone that reminded me of his mood when I told him many years ago there was no Santa Claus.

"I'm fumbling for the right words here, but … ahh, I've been having serious memory problems for some time," I said.

"What's up, Dad?" he asked candidly, focused on the road and what may lay ahead.

"Well, I've been getting lost often, confused about the time and place, my judgment has been lacking at times, I'm having difficulties problem solving, and experiencing much rage. Kinda like Gam, you know."

"What do the doctors say?" he asked. "No bullshit, Dad. What's up?"

"It's not the final act I was expecting at this stage in life," I said. "I thought I'd bow out more gracefully. But recently, I've had a batch of clinical tests and a brain scan."

"So what's up, Dad?" he asked again, more to the point.

"I've just been diagnosed with early-onset Alzheimer's," I told him.

Brendan kept driving, his eyes fixed on the road. He was absorbing, then finally said, "That explains a lot."

He, like others, had noticed the early symptoms, but passed it off as my eccentricities—creativity—over time. We talked about it for several miles; he asked questions about the diagnosis, what it meant, and about the future for both me and the family. Brendan had more questions; I was getting uneasy with the conversation, thinking about the classic Jon Lovitz line in the movie *City Slickers*, "Too much information!" I shut down. So we drove on, talking about other things, the usual father/son stuff—work, sports, and politics of the day. Brendan reinforced his love and full support, but was predictably guarded in emotion as he digested the conversation—a shield he would drop soon.

****

I was looking forward weeks later to a July 4th weekend trip to bucolic Coronado Island off San Diego, trying not to focus on seminal moments in my life that all seemed to be happening near Independence Day. Coronado, five miles off the port of San Diego, is a paradise of a place—an out-of-body, other world experience, a place where one can forget.

But first there was unfinished business. I had to speak with the other kids. I learned early on in journalism that if you don't tell your story, someone else will tell it for you. That wouldn't have been right here.

My daughter, Colleen, was on the Cape on a short break from her duties in Washington, D.C. as a communications analyst on contract with Homeland Security. She now teaches underprivileged kids in a Baltimore elementary school. Conor, a junior at the time, studying sports management at Johnson & Wales University in Providence, was hanging at the house. So, we asked Brendan to come down from Boston for a family conference, under the guise that we'd all go to dinner, which eventually we did—a great meal at Joe's Tavern in East Orleans, a local family hangout on the way to Nauset Beach.

I've always been late, and this time was no exception, as the kids waited with inevitable annoyance for me in the living room, as I contemplated in earshot in my bathroom what I was about to tell them. My ears were burning. I was looking for the right words.

"So, anyone want a drink?" I asked, as I finally emerged.

"Daaaaad, let's get going," Colleen said, with nodding assurance from Brendan and Conor. "It's getting late."

"I'm having a glass of red wine. Who wants one?" I said in yet another attempt at delay.

The kids, eyes rolling, obliged. My wife, knowing the script, already had hers in hand. Maybe a double or a triple.

"Your father has something to tell you," she prompted me.

All eyes were in my direction. Stage fright has never been an issue for me, but the words were not flowing, as I was accustomed in life. *Get to the freakin' point*, I thought, assuming that Brendan might already have passed some of our conversation along to his siblings.

It was an awkward talk, one couched with language that explained the diagnosis, the need for the family to buckle up, but left hope in the room. There were questions, tears, and hugs. I think, at some level, they all knew. No one really wanted to talk about it. Finally, Conor broke the ice, as the youngest of the family can often do.

"So, Dad, you're losing your mind!" he said.

"You might say so," I replied.

We all laughed; there was no comeback. We all seemed to understand. Now, on to dinner and talk of the Patriots, Red Sox, Celtics, Bruins, Pluto, and the Milky Way. Life goes on, as Robert Frost said, particularly if we seek to move forward; times to share, bills to pay. Woody Allen in a wry exchange in the movie *Annie Hall* put an exclamation point on survival instincts in an anecdote about a guy who goes to a psychiatrist, complaining about his brother who thinks he's a chicken. When the doctor suggests he turn his brother in, the man replies, "I would, but I need the eggs!"

My family needs the eggs.

****

The flight to San Diego was peaceful; departing Boston and flying high above the jagged harbor islands, I tried to leave my baggage behind. I've always been captivated, flying coast to coast, watching this magnificent country unfold beneath me. Good thinking weather. Hours later, as the plane banked a right over the Pacific Ocean to line up with a runway, I felt cleansed. But as the great Roman Empire scribe Publius Flavius Vegetius Renatus cautioned centuries ago, "In time of peace, prepare for war!"

Coronado, connected to San Diego by a ten-mile isthmus called the Silver Strand, offers some of the nation's finest beaches and enough natural beauty and gawking potential to satisfy the most judicious traveler. Spanish for "the crowned one," Coronado is a jewel of an isle. I couldn't wait.

The first night, Brendan, my brother-in-law, Louie, and I stayed at the Coronado Island Marriott Resort, overlooking the pristine San Diego Bay and the downtown. My wife, who had arrived earlier, spent the evening at the Hotel del Coronado with her sister, Nancy, who had been named in my will as special family medical consultant; I knew Nancy would always have my best interest at heart, and wouldn't dispatch me prematurely to a nursing home.

After a late afternoon swim, a fresh fish dinner, and a walk along the boardwalk, Brendan, Lou, and I went back to the hotel. Lou, a great guy, but a lard ass of a night owl, wanted to go to bed again, so Brendan and I walked to a bar for a beer. There was still some unfinished business between us. He had no clue. Timing can be terrible, particularly on a flee from reality; it often has no respect for timelines.

I had brought with me all the signed legal documents naming Brendan as my power of attorney and my legal guardian, should something ever happen to Mary Catherine. All assets, if anything left, would pass to him to be distributed to the kids. I was to have nothing, just as the lawyers wanted. Brendan needed to know this. Now was the time. Timing often sucks, even on placid Coronado.

Once again, I couldn't find the right words over a Blue Moon, even with a slice of orange on the lip of a chilled glass. So, we walked back to the hotel and I engaged him in conversation on the second floor balcony outside our room, above what seemed to be a plantation of palms and tropical flowers, sifting in the sultry Coronado ocean breeze.

I showed him the documents. He wanted nothing to do with it. Nothing.

"I don't want to talk about it!" he shouted. *"I don't want to fucking talk about it!"*

"But you gotta," I said. "You have to know, Brendan. We have to talk. You're the oldest boy and you have to start acting like it. I need you. Get it!"

It was the most powerful confrontation I've ever had with

any of my children, one I hope never to repeat.

I showed him the documents again. He pushed them away. *"This is bullshit! It's fucking bullshit!"* he screamed.

"Fine, then you need to see something else," I replied, opening the door to the hotel room to bring out another pile of papers. They were my medical records, a word picture of a swan dive off a cliff.

"Read 'em," I said, waving the papers in front of his face. "Look at them. They're right here!"

We were both in rage. My brother-in-law woke up, poked his head out to the balcony, and asked if everything was all right.

"It's fine, Lou," I said, motioning him quickly back into the room.

Brendan grabbed the papers, about 30 pages in all, and began to read.

He stopped at a page that summarized the neurologist's finding.

"The diagnosis has been made in my opinion," the doctor's report said. " ... I am not sure how much longer he has in terms of being able to reliably and meaningfully provide the quality of work he has put out in the past. It may also be helpful if his counselor would help in negotiating more open discussion of his growing limitations with other family members so he suffers less isolation."

Brendan was stunned.

"This is bullshit! This is bullshit!" he yelled in a voice that pierced within.

In primal anger, he ripped the documents into pieces, then tossed them off the balcony. The chunks of paper—my personal, naked, and wrenching medical reports—fell among the palms like a blanket of snow.

"This is bullshit! That's what I think. It's bullshit!" he yelled even louder, his eyes now tearing up.

He paused for a second to catch his breath. "It's bullshit,

Dad. It's just fucking BULLSHIT!" He stopped again, sobbed, and then said in a lowered voice, "It's bullshit because I know it's true!"

He then fell into my arms and cried like a baby. We hugged, talked some more, and then went to bed.

I didn't sleep well that night. I awoke at first light to the realization, the horror, that my medical records—documentation that I was losing my mind, as Conor had pointed out days earlier—were strewn among paradise, all throughout the tropical plants, near the pool.

I grabbed a plastic trash bag, and picked up as many pieces of the clinical reports, test results, and medical comments as I could. My past and my future were now in the trash.

6

The Wayback Machine

Mister Peabody was the smartest beagle ever to walk the Earth. Everyone over 55 knows this. In cartoon terms, he was an inventor, entrepreneur, scientist, Nobel Laureate, and a two-time Olympic medalist. Impressive for a member of the humble hound group.

Appearing in the late 1950s and early '60s, as the erudite canine of *Rocky and His Friends* and *The Bullwinkle Show*, Mister Peabody, in benevolence, adopted a dorky, orange-haired orphan named Sherman. In a moment of dog genius, Mr. Peabody invented the "WABAC" machine as a birthday gift for his surrogate "son," a rejiggered "should-have-been-machine," in modern culture often referred to as the Wayback Machine, a convenient way to reintroduce issues or events of the past, as we would like to view them.

I suspect Mister Peabody in his self-referential humor might have had early-onset Alzheimer's; yet, he was a virtuoso in his day. I find that Mr. Peabody's WABAC Machine, a time tunnel, has greater relevance in some ways than reality *du jour*.

My life today has become a cartoon in so many ways, a Wayback Machine, but the early years give me ballast.

****

Way back, my late maternal grandmother, Brooklyn-born Loretta Sinnott Brown, called me "snippy snooper" as a young boy because I was always "snooping around," asking too many questions, forever wanting to know the minutia of life. She and my maternal grandfather, George Walter Brown—born in Manhattan, an earnest man who had owned several Upper East Side brownstones and munificently forgave missed rents during the Depression with a heart of the size of SoHo—lived on Rye Beach Avenue in Rye, N.Y. in a classic red brick two-story home, a short walk from Rye Beach on Long Island Sound at the mouth of New York Harbor. My grandparents had grown up in the city, worked there, then made their way north, as with all my relatives, maternal and paternal, since kin began arriving generations ago from the old sod, from places like Dublin, Wexford, County Clare, and Belfast.

My grandfather, whom we affectionately called "Daddy George," had close ties to Magherafelt, Ireland in the Northern Ireland County of Derry where family members were baptized and married in the Little Chapel of Woods, which still stands today, framed by a family burial marker.

Once or twice a week, my mother used to take me and two of my sisters, Maureen and Lauren, to see my grandmother and Daddy George. Grandma was petite, short, and thin, a woman of incalculable resolve—perseverance that she clearly passed down to my mother. Daddy George was handsome, gentle, and erudite, an intellectual in his day—small in stature, large in bounty. He didn't talk much, as we observed as kids; Grandma did all the chatting, distracting us with sandwiches and desserts, piping hot chocolate in winter in a tall steaming glass, and in summer, fresh lemonade and blackberries from the back yard. I spent much time with her in the kitchen, snooping around and playing with her dog, a Mexican Chihuahua named Poncho, appropriate in dimension for the household. Mom, meanwhile, sat on the couch visiting with her dad, trying to make conversation. The moment seemed awkward.

In time, I began to realize that something was terribly wrong with my grandfather. His sentences were becoming shorter as his voice trailed off. He didn't recognize us on occasion, and he stared a lot in withdrawal. Often, he just shook his head, in an acknowledgment when asked a question. I thought he was hard of hearing.

There were times, my mother told me later, when Daddy George in great confusion would walk to the Rye train station without telling anyone, taking an express to Grand Central so he could stroll the streets of the Upper East Side—a place that made him feel whole. He was trying to go home to his office on 28th Street. The local New York cops knew him and would phone my grandmother, then make sure he returned safely. No one seemed to grasp what was happening.

Daddy George, doctors said, had "hardening of the arteries," the cipher in those days for dementia. "Your grandfather is very sick," Mom would tell us.

I'll never forget the day we came for a visit, and all the dining room furniture, including the mahogany table on which I had done my grammar school homework, was gone—replaced with a stark hospital bed. Daddy George could no longer walk up the steep oak stairs and was confined to the bed.

The deterioration had a solemn impact on me. My grandfather, who had been slowly waning before us, was now in a deep slide—in the rear-view mirror of Grandma, who cared for him like a trained nurse; my mother, who adored him for all he was; and my siblings and me, who felt the pull of a family tree. We loved him. A photograph of Daddy George, sepia in tone, in a suit and tie in his professional Manhattan days, hangs in my office today; it's the same photograph that I hung on a wall at the foot of my mom's bed at EPOCH Senior Living in Brewster, months before she succumbed to Alzheimer's. The night before she passed away, I pointed at the photo, and my mother recognized him. With his wire-rimmed glasses and the shape of his face, I look a bit like him.

Weeks before my grandfather died, Grandma on her loving rounds, was stunned one day to see Daddy George sitting up in bed. He spoke for the first time in months, and said in muted tones that he was aware of all she had done for him; he thanked her, and told her that he loved her. It was a last expression of love—testimony that those suffering from dementia and other mental handicaps, still observe and can retain far more than one might imagine. My mom rushed over to the house to speak with her dad. Doctors counseled that the enlightenment was fleeting, a last flow of blood to the brain or a remnant brain cell flashing a final distress signal. Daddy George quickly fell back into the abyss.

I will never forget the day he died. Still haunts me. When I returned to the red brick house, the hospital bed was gone and the dining room furniture was back in place, as if nothing had happened, yet I knew that nothing would ever be the same.

****

Nothing ever is the same, beyond history that repeats itself. "No man ever steps in the same river twice," the Greek philosopher Heraclitus of Ephesus wrote in 500 BC, "for it's not the same river, and he's not the same man . . . Other waters are forever flowing on to you."

In Alzheimer's, the currents of the disease rise slowly. Those with early-onset, with an acuity of what's to come, hold a collective breath, awaiting progressions of the loss. "Oh waste of loss," Thomas Wolfe, one of my favorite writers, observed in his 1929 novel, *Look Homeward Angel*, "Remembering speechlessly we seek the great forgotten language, the lost lane into Heaven, a stone, a leaf, a door. Where? When?"

The where and when is always front of mind with me. When my grandfather chased the forgotten language in Alzheimer's, he was lost cerebrally in a back alley; he never found it. Grandfather was never the same again, yet my mother rarely spoke of his illness, other than to say that he had suffered greatly, but with inspiring dignity. That's the way one should suffer, she told me. Always suffer with great dignity. Later, when my mother was diagnosed with Alzheimer's, family members were equally voiceless about the illness, in sync with denial, reacting to a stigma—a common antiphon to Alzheimer's and other life-changing diseases. Myself included.

"It's not denial," once observed cartoonist Bill Watterson, creator of the precocious, at times sardonic, comic strip *Calvin and Hobbes*. "I'm just selective about the reality I accept."

Aren't we all . . .

****

More than one in three today (far more in years to come) are touched in some way by the disease—either fighting it, or knowing a family member, colleague, or friend with Alzheimer's—and yet, the disease rarely gets attention in an obituary or in a death certificate. Family members often decline even to acknowledge Alzheimer's, or call it by name. This collective denial has been the subject of scores of newspaper, magazine, and medical journal commentaries. "Scientists say that when they try to trace the inheritance of Alzheimer's disease in family members, or to learn the age of onset, they come up against family members who will not admit that a parent or close relative had anything seriously wrong with them," noted *The New York Times* years ago in a report. "Adult children frequently try to protect their parents by not telling them that they have Alzheimer's disease, a situation reminiscent of the days when no one would tell cancer patients that they had cancer . . . The stigma, experts say, is because of the disturbing symptoms and the fears of family members that they could inherit a gene that will give them the disease."

And so, family members across the board often reach, explicably, for a shallow, "drive-by" diagnosis after a brief encounter or a hasty phone conversation. It's fully human to deny what we find unpleasant or chilling, but when the drive-by precludes one from the facts, from facing real-life implications, then it's wholly unproductive, a dead end.

Such observations are akin to saying to one who cannot hear: "But you don't look like you're deaf."

****

You can't hear much on Pluto. It's a dark icy place, dense with denial, isolated to the point of impenetrable peace. What's in a name? Plenty, in this case. In 1930, Walt Disney introduced an obtuse canine companion for Mickey Mouse named Pluto, an apparent callout to a planet with a thin atmosphere of nitrogen, methane, and carbon monoxide gases, the kind of place in deep space of suspended animation where not much cohesive thought occurs. Beyond Pluto, three times farther from Earth and 900 times Earth's distance from the Sun, is Sedna, a surface composition of 60 percent of methane ice and 70 percent of water ice; it is capable of supporting a subsurface ocean of liquid water, scientists say. This dwarf planet will become closer and brighter over the next 72 years before it begins its 10,500-year trip to the far reaches of the solar system and back again, making it much easier for some to hop on a ride from Pluto, a sling shot. You can hear God from here.

The trip to Pluto, a metaphor of survival instinct for my

flight from reality, can be a comfort, a release from the angst, fear, sadness, and rage—a surrender to numbness, those un-fathomable blank stares, to feel peaceful again, avoid the pain of losing control. Daily, I fight against the impulse to let go, a welcome release, even just for minutes. There are days I have to prompt myself to come back. Often, my wife, children, or friends summon me with a snap of a finger.

The drifting is similar to sailing in a slack wind. In Alzhei-mer's, one doesn't move fast, but the journey is soporific—respite from the interruptions of a brain gone awry, a flickering light whose plug is loose in the socket. On Pluto, the mind and body are at peace, no longer on high alert. The metaphoric gravita-tional pull of Pluto, for me and others with the disease, draws deep. It's soothing at this stage just to let go. At some point, the light goes dark forever.

Often, I look, with soulful flashlight in hand, for my mother on Pluto, but I know she's not there. She's with God. Many months ago, one evening when I couldn't sleep, typical of my journey, I was lying late at night on the couch in the family room, watching reruns of "Planet Earth." I sensed a woman sit-ting next to me. I wasn't sure if I had drifted off, was in-between sleep, or was just dreaming. Still not sure. At first, I thought it was my wife, Mary Catherine; her back was to me. Then the woman turned and looked at me. It was my mother. She stared straight at me.

"Mom," I said. "I can't sleep!"

"It's ok. I can't sleep either," she replied in a calming tone.

From what I recall from the encounter, she then rubbed the back of my head, and within seconds, I fell into a deep slumber. It was the most restful, peaceful sleep of a lifetime.

My mother in time would make her presence known else-where, once in the form, I suspect, of a flowering hibiscus. My sister Lauren had received a hibiscus from a friend, but the plant would only flower on rare occasions, remarkably rare occurrences and in yellow: on my mom's birthday and when family gathered at Lauren's outside Boston. As if to reinforce like the elementary teacher she was, my mother's presence was felt again. Driving down to the Cape on a summer day shortly after my mom's death, Lauren spotted a yellow jeep as she queued up for gas along Pilgrims Highway. Her attention was fixed on the license plate, surrounded by a sea of yellow. It read: "RIP Mom."

Rest in peace, always.

These types of happenstance are daring to attest; one opens themselves up to all sorts of second-guessing. I get that. So analyze away.

Yet, on a cold January night a year later, I was sleeping on the couch again, my wife was in the throes of a horrific sinus infection. I got up, as I do every two hours, just to walk around the house, often aimlessly. This time, I had to take another pee, and on the way back to the couch, I checked the digital clock on the stove. It was 4:12 am, still dark, black as night. As I walked to the couch, I noticed something moving slowly to port side of the wood stove where embers were alight. It was an image of sorts, but instinctively, I was serene with it. At first, I thought it was just another visual misperception, or as we scribes might correctly call it, another hallucination. I was wide awake at the time, focusing intensely on the image. I saw the outline of a woman. She had blonde hair, dressed in clothing familiar to me. The image moved slowly toward me, then backward, then toward me again. The woman was beckoning me with her right hand to follow. She kept summoning. I realized then it was my mother, or a likeness of her. The shadows of a man stood behind. Slowly, she summoned to him, as she had with me, to move forward. I wondered if it was my father. The image in the shadow hesitated, and I thought in the moment that if any of this were real, my father was probably saying to Mom, "Ginny, let's not scare the shit out of Greg!"

I was at peace, but it wasn't my time to move forward. So, I turned on a light. Saw nothing. I turned it off. Saw nothing. Then I went back to bed in great calm, intuitively feeling that I wasn't alone. I told my wife about the experience the following day. I joked with her that my mother was looking for one of her recipes. I want to believe it was my mother, but what if it wasn't? What terrifies me is yet another manifestation of this disease.

7

Smart Pills

S LEEP IS GOOD FOR THE SOUL, BUT WAKING HOURS
are when work gets done, with the brain in the "on" position. Whatever one's aspiration in life, an engaged brain is fully
focused with vigorous mentoring. Among great tutors in my life,
I had exceptional coaches in high school at Archbishop Stepinac
High School (class of 1968) on Mamaroneck Avenue in White
Plains, five exits up Route 95 from the Bronx. I had a passion
for sports, but enjoyed the expression of theater and turned to
the stage. Drama coaches Father James Cashman and Father
Bernie McMahon were particularly inspiring, instructing to
express, yet stay within, to never show fear, to ad lib in a manner
that always built confidence. They were lifelong teachers. Two of
their prized students went on to far greater successes—Academy
Award winning actor Jon Voight, class of 1956, and Alan Alda,

class of 1952, of "MASH" fame and other generational movies. But the actor I seem to emulate most these days is the late
Lenny Montana, who played Luca Brasi, the dim hitman in *The
Godfather*. My favorite scene is Luca Brasi's reprised, slow slur,
preparing himself for a wedding salutation to Don Corleone,
just to get it right.

"Don Corleone, I am honored and grateful that you have
invited me to your home on the wedding day of your daughter.
And may their first child be a masculine child," Brasi kept prac-
ticing in a slow, deliberate, and discomfited pace.

Before business meetings these days, before every family
gathering, every outreach, every salutation, I rehearse my lines,
just to get them straight. I prep for the quips, the thoughtful
commentaries, and salutations. I study the lines. Sometimes, I
keep crib notes. Nothing is ever left to chance these days. Then,
it's showtime! I'm pretty good at it; damn good, in fact. Fathers
Cashman and McMahon taught me well—teachers who trained
me with great insight, humility, and faith in one's ability to
row harder.

You have to row harder with dementia, or you drift. In the
sport of crew, with roots dating back to ancient Egyptian times,
you must work as a team, propelling the racing shell through
churning waters. But in Alzheimer's, one must pull an oar with
the strength of a strokeman, only there is no one else in the shell
for the "catch" and "recovery." At the catch, a rower's hips are
aligned with the oarlock for maximum thrust of the blade in
the water. The rower then applies pressure to the oar by pushing the seat toward the bow by extension of the legs. As the
legs approach a full extension, the rower pivots the torso toward
the bow, and then finally pulls the arms toward the chest. The
hands meet the chest right above the diaphragm, and then drop
enough to take the blade out of the water. At the very end of the
stroke, with the blade still in the water, the hands drop slightly
to unload the oar so that spring energy stored in the bend of

the oar gets transferred to the boat. This eases removing the oar from the water and minimizes energy wasted on lifting water above the surface in splashing.

The recovery phase follows the drive—removing the oar from the water and coordinating the body movement to move the oar to the catch again.

And so it is with Alzheimer's—a catch and recovery to engage a brain on its way to deluge.

Sure, there are many who encourage from the shoreline: family, friends, doctors, and colleagues, many of them not fully understanding why they are waving. In Alzheimer's, one is in the boat alone. So, you row a little harder!

****

Dementia today comes in many flavors, a cornucopia of medical terms. Old-style labels like "hardening of the arteries" have given way to a more technical lexicon. Now there are more than 80 types of dementias identified. Alzheimer's is the most prevalent; others include: Lewy body dementia, Creutzfeldt-Jakob disease, Huntington disease, frontal or temporal lobe dementias (including Pick's disease and Primary progressive aphasia), HIV-associated dementia, Dementia pugilistica (Boxer's Syndrome), Corticobasal degeneration, and other genetically related dementias.

The progression of Alzheimer's can be slowed, to some extent, with state-of-the art prescriptions used to diffuse symptoms, producing "decoy" chemicals that trick enzymes that break down the transmitter chemical (acetylcholine), allowing it to perform as well as it can. I take a daily cocktail of drugs. The combination dosage helps slow the rate of decline on good days. The Aricept (donepezil) works to improve the function of the nerve cells by slowing a breakdown of the transmitter chemical acetylcholine. Namenda (memantine hcl) assists in blocking transmission of chemicals in the brain that kills nerve cells.

Close friends call them my "smart pills!"

Consider the 1982 movie *Tron* where a computer programmer is transported inside the software world of a computer mainframe and engages terrifying sequencers in an effort to get back. That's my world today, and the destiny of millions of others, unless something is done to subdue the insidious intruder.

****

The mornings for me are always the same. In disarray. At first light, I must focus on the five Ws: the who, what, where, when, why, and how of life, as if rebooting my faithful MacBook Pro before tossing the covers and organizing the scattered files of my mind. I do it out of instinct, but there's always the depression, fear, and angst to walk through, and that's just on the way to the bathroom where, on doctors' advice, I've begun labeling the toothpaste, liquid soap, and rubbing alcohol. I have attempted often to brush my teeth with liquid soap, and on two occasions gargled briefly with rubbing alcohol. Scope is far better!

Then, I go deep into my lists—notes for everything, printed and on my iPhone calendar with repeat advisories. My life has become a strategy. I have a playbook, a script, backup for everything. Sometimes, the stratagem is just showing up, other times it's deflection; more often, it's an ongoing quest for excellence, understanding as best as possible the new boundaries. I have a formidable enemy—my mind. It used to be my best friend. I don't see any chance now for reconciliation. *Illegitimi non carborundum*, as I say: don't let the bastards grind you down.

Cartoonist Gary Larson always got right to the point. A classic 1986 image underscores a debate over whether the brain can expand. In Larson's illustration, a student with a bulky frame and a particularly tiny head, raises his left hand in a crowded classroom. The clock on the back wall reads 10 am. "Mr. Osborne," the caption reads, "may I be excused? My brain is full."

Clinically, our brains are never full, but there are days when I feel mine is empty. The eerie image of novelist Jack Torrance in the Stanley Kubrick chiller, *The Shining*, haunts me—Torrance, played by a young Jack Nicholson, working his manuscript to the point of madness in a whiteout of a blizzard at the deserted Overlook Hotel, drafting horrifying pages and pages: "All work and no play makes Jack a dull boy."

The play for me is a daily exercise of body and mind to engage the brain, as if pulling the chord to a cold chainsaw. You gotta rip at it, attempting at least to understand how the brain works. Some say the brain acts as a computer; others suggest it's a symphony orchestra. The brain is probably a little of both, perhaps more of an orchestra with various sections that must execute on cue for bravado of a performance. Hence tune-ups of mind, body, and spirit are critical to the process.

So at twilight, I'm back on the mat with the monster. That's why I run several miles each night to increase the cerebral flow as the sun sets, and more confusion takes over; I run until my legs give out. Due to my recent diagnosis and pain of acute spinal stenosis and scoliosis, I'm unable to run as I did, so now I crank the treadmill at the gym each night to an elevation of 15 at a speed of up to 6.2, and race walk four to five miles. The pain is still present, though there is less pounding on the spinal cord. My daily physical routine helps reduce end-of-day confusion and restlessness, common in dementia patients and known as "sundowning," caused as light fades to black. This can be a time of greater rage, agitation, and mood swings, much like dandelions that behave differently at night; their heads close up tightly as the sun goes down.

On doctors' orders, I try vigorously to exercise my body and mind every night. After the gym, I usually write for two hours. Medical experts encourage those with Alzheimer's and other forms of dementia to pursue the creative arts, particularly writ- ers, musicians, and artists with the disease. The writing makes me feel whole again—until the confusion takes over.

In Alzheimer's, mental and physical fatigue increases, and the restlessness can lead to pacing or wandering because an individual can't sleep. Theorists say that with the development of plaques and tangles in the brain related to Alzheimer's, there may be a disruption at sunset in what doctors term the "suprachiasmatic nucleus," associated with sleep patterns and changes in lighting—bringing on a sundowning effect.

With this disease, the sun rises and sets on a foggy bottom, a haze at times that precludes one, among other things, from recognizing familiar faces; or worse yet, the disease transposes a face, like the 1997 action thriller, *Face/Off*, starring Nicolas Cage and John Travolta. My life now, it seems, is a series of anecdotes. In Alzheimer's, there are times when one sees and experiences things that are not real, and times when one can't distinguish people and places that are.

There have been mornings when I haven't recognized my wife lying next to me. I knew I was supposed to be in the bed with this attractive woman, but I wasn't sure who she was. She looked familiar, but I had no understanding for several minutes of my relationship with the woman I have slept with for 37 years. It is disturbing; I never let on to her about the shame of it. She was asleep, so I just let it go.

And then there was the time at Kennedy Airport in New York in November 2010, awaiting my brother-in-law, Carl Maresca, and two of my brothers, Tim and Andy, for a flight to Shannon on an annual visit to Ireland, a place that restores the thinker and writer in me.

We were flying into Shannon to tour again the bucolic West Coast, a place that has attracted writers and artists for centuries, from Dingle to Donegal with its tiered cliffs, surging green pastures framed with moss-covered stonewalls, and snug, mottled villages that inspire poetry. From there, we were to hop a train cross-island to Dublin to take in this magnificent ancient city at the confluence of the River Liffey and the Irish Sea, a city that traces its beginnings back to 140 AD and claims among its sons James Joyce, William Butler Yates, and Samuel Beckett.

Sitting at the gate at Kennedy, I thought in long-term memory about walks through Trinity College, founded in 1592, along O'Connell Street, the site of the 1916 Easter Rising, the War of Irish Independence, and the Temple Bar, *Barra an Teampaill* in Gaelic, an area on the south bank of the Liffey. This cultural, and yes, pub district, likely received its name from the Temple family, who lived here in the 17th century; Sir William Temple was provost of Trinity College in 1609. In the core of the Temple Bar is Fishamble Street—the site of the first performance of Handel's *Messiah* on April 12, 1742; the annual performance of the *Messiah* is held on the same date at the same location. At a nearby tavern on Eustace Street in 1791, the republican revolutionary group, the Society of the United Irishmen, was formed. The group launched the Irish Rebellion of 1798 in an effort to end British rule over Ireland and to create an independent Irish Republic. In a maze of narrow, cobblestone streets, the Temple Bar captures the spirit of Dublin.

I'd rather muse on history than reality—the past is more redeeming to me than the future. It is a place of peace. My daze, call it reverie, was interrupted by a tap on the back.

"Hey, Lunchie!"

I earned the moniker "free lunch" years ago from my father because of my penchant for a free lunch, handouts from the nuns, and anyone with a basket.

"Hey, Lunchie!" the man called out again.

I stared at him intently, and didn't know him. I was getting pissed that this man in his 60s was calling me "Lunchie." New Yorkers are always in your face.

"You ok?" the stranger inquired.

Do I know you from Pluto? I wondered.

I stared at him again, carefully studying his expression, then began to connect the dots. The mosaic slowly resonated with familiarity. I focused in again. It was my brother-in-law Carl—a first-generation Italian American with Solarino roots. I've known him from the second grade; we attended Resurrection Catholic School in Rye, he has always been an older brother to me, and always has my back.

"I'm your legal guardian on this trip," he said with a smile. "So shape up! We're going to make you wear a sandwich board with a phone number on the back of it; if you get lost, people will know who to call."

Gotta love those Italians! And I do. They are the salt of the Earth, with a little oregano on the side.

****

Not far beyond the bend of Doanes Creek in Harwich on the Cape, back on the lip of Nantucket Sound at the mouth of stately Wychmere Harbor—a full circle of geologic perfection—is the confluence of all that is Cape Cod.

At the entrance to the harbor, marked by a sturdy stone jetty, is a graceful wide swath of sandy beach, one of the few accreting beaches on the Cape and growing at a rate of up to seven feet a year, given the steady ebb and flow of littoral currents.

Inside the harbor to the north is a row of sleek sailboards and pleasure craft in summer, guarding like sentinels on watch the comings and goings of the channel and overlooking the site of the legendary Thompson's Clam Bar, once one of the largest seasonal seafood restaurants east of the Mississippi. It served some of the finest clams known to man. Patrons would wait up to an hour-and-a-half for a table in the 450-seat waterview restaurant, turning out more than 2,000 seafood dinners on a hot July night.

The venerable structure is now the cornerstone of the exclusive Wychmere Beach Club in Harwich Port, a luxury private club.

On cue the afternoon of Sunday, June 19, 2011, the beach club's opening, the sun was glistening high above Nantucket Sound. My job as a media consultant was to lure the press and work the crowd over pricey Chardonnay and Cabernet and an assortment of fresh seafood and a raw bar that you would find at the finest New York and Boston bistros. I do nice work, arriving fashionably late, but on cue, and dressed in Tommy Bahama chinos, saddle shoes, and a shirt I bought in Dublin that looked like it was right off the deck of the Titanic. No assembly instructions required on this assignment, I assumed. Everything was perfect. Even my good buddy, John Piekarski, was there, standing by the pool with a handful of oysters and chatting up the elite. John hadn't told me he was coming.

I interrupted his conversation with a definitive pat on the back. "This guy boring you?" I asked.

The cold stares, even from John, could have frozen my retinas, only it wasn't John. It was a high roller from the city, not the kind of guy who appreciated a slap on the back and a stab in the shoulder from a less-than-perfect stranger. I finally realized all this after standing inelegantly next to the man for about a minute. With dots in the brain reconnecting, it wasn't even close. This guy didn't even look like John now.

So, I did my best Roseanne Roseannadanna of SNL fame, the character perfected by Gilda Radner: "Well, never mind."

"My mistake," I apologized. "Sorry!"

I walked away, feeling a pulse in my throbbing head.

It was the first time I had such an extraterrestrial experience. I have known John Piekarski for 30 years. I immediately thought of my mother and the times she had such disconnects. The realization was deadening. I moved on. All was good now, so I thought. When you fall off a horse you get right back on. Time to start up another conversation, I reasoned.

"You probably don't know me," I said minutes later to another gentleman standing near a walkway that led to the beach.

I reached out my hand. He shook it, and laughed.

"Funny!" the guy said, shaking his head.

How did I go from being an idiot to a funny man in the space of a few minutes, I wondered?

I looked at him closely, stared intently. No recognition.

"Sorry I didn't get right back to you after our meeting the other day," the man apologized.

The deadness was upon me again. Like the dutiful student, I started asking questions, trying to fill in the blanks, stitching together a story. Something. A clue that would give me direction, edification. Nothing. The mind was blank.

I pursued a line of conversation and questioning, with a reporter's instinct—small talk about sports and the summer ahead. Don't panic, stay in the moment, never let on. As Roman Emperor and stoic philosopher Marcus Aurelius advised in the first century, "Confine yourself to the present." I've employed this strategy for years; it's a wait-and-see approach until I can either make a connection or exit the conversation gracefully.

"Greg, I want you to meet a friend," he said of the man to his left. "I think you can help him in his business."

Both had their business cards out on a table. Finally, a clue. *Shit.* I realized then that I was in conversation with a close client I had known for years and whose wife is a friend of mine.

Coming full circle, I suppose the silver lining in Alzheimer's, if you're good on your feet, and even if you're not, you get to meet new friends daily.

****

I would have that chance to meet new friends again months later at a consultant meeting at Gillette Stadium in Foxboro where I've been a consultant to the Kraft Group for years, working in areas of community outreach and communications strategies. I arrived early for a meeting with Scott Farmelant, a friend and fellow consultant, a principal of the Boston communication firm Mills Public Relations. Months earlier, I had confided in him about my Alzheimer's diagnosis, as doctors had suggested with close clients and consultants. We discussed future projects and Scott's willingness to help fill in the blanks outside of my protected box of writing and communication skills. It was a business arrangement, born out of friendship and Scott's empathy for the progressive disease.

I was a bit out of sorts that day, but covering myself in the best reportorial spin. Some of the dots, as they often do unannounced, weren't connecting. I had been off my medication for a day or two—simply forgot to take it. But I was determined to fight through the haze on this brilliant sunny January day.

As I entered the room, I didn't recognize anyone; they looked vaguely familiar, but assumed a new crew of campaign workers had moved in. A guy to my left, a friendly, enthusiastic individual, started chatting me up about the campaign.

We talked about project benefits, opposition issues, media, and messaging. He clearly knew me, but I was embarrassed to ask who he was.

"Let's go grab some coffee," he said after some chat.

"That's good with me," I said, "but I'm waiting for Scott Farmelant, then we can all go."

There was silence.

The guy put his arm around me and whispered into my ear, "Greg, I'm Scott!"

Altogether mortified, but not off my humor game, I replied, "Well then, that's good, Scott. Now we don't have to wait for you."

We walked out of the room for coffee on a one-two count, and never spoke about the disconnect again. Scott's a good friend.

8

Rocks in My Head

Dr. seuss once advised, "you've got brains in your head. You have and feet in your shoes. You can steer yourself in any direction you choose."

Not if you have rocks in your head.

Since I was a boy, my mother said I had rocks in my head; now after decades, they are literally calcifying, obstructing signals to the brain. Early-onset Alzheimer's will do that.

I've always been a good rainmaker, the art of inducing precipitation, in this case, generating puddles for the family to pay bills, but of late, the signals are crossing. While I was never an exemplary steward, I'm spending money today in odd ways, at times like a drunken sailor. At doctors' directive, I've turned all my credit cards over to my wife, who along with my faithful sister Lauren, an accountant-type, views all my online bank and debit-card statements daily to make sure nothing is awry. Surprises were occurring regularly, until I was forced to hand over a hidden American Express card I had kept to maintain a sense of self.

The final straw was Christmas 2011. I'm a Clark Griswold, "Sparky" dad; each Christmas Eve after church service, the family has an intimate dinner at the Chatham Bars Inn, overlooking Chatham's inner harbor, then we ceremoniously watch Chevy Chase's *Christmas Vacation*. We still laugh so hard we cry—aping all the iconic lines seconds before they are delivered.

I usually go overboard for Christmas, akin to Evil Knievel attempting to jump the Grand Canyon on a revved up motorcycle. This particular Christmas was no exception in holiday largesse, but early that Christmas Eve was a moment of unusual stillness for me, the cerebral kind. Listening to *Silent Night* on a speaker outsider a retail store at noon, I was flush suddenly with the fear that I had no gifts, that everyone else in the family had gone Christmas shopping but me. I began to panic. So, I whipped out the American Express Gold, and within 15 minutes bought close to a thousand dollars of stuff that I had no recollection of buying—the kind of crap nobody wants: shot glasses with Boston Celtic logos, paper plates and plastic forks, a doormat. I wrapped the "presents" like a good elf, placed them under the tree, and awaited Christmas morning.

To my horror, on Christmas morning, I realized that I had bought the mother lode weeks earlier, nice presents actually, and when it came time to open my inane offerings of late, I first got stares from my wife and kids, some humiliating laughs, a few loving cautions, and then a big hand from son Brendan—asking for the American Express card so that everything could be returned for a credit.

Talk about pissing your money away. I hope you kids see what a silly waste of resources this was, my wife must have thought in her best impersonation of Clark's mother-in-law after he had placed

250 strands of lights with 100 bulbs on each strand for a total of 25,000 light bulbs on the house, and none of them worked.

If I woke up tomorrow with my head sewn to the carpet, I wouldn't be more surprised, I thought.

****

Like the Griswold house, the lights in my head blink; they are full on, off, back on, then off again, on again. Sometimes, I can sense it coming; other times, I can't—the disconnects, dropped calls, mental pocket dials, short-term memory losses, and the tingling of the mind, which starts like an ocean swell in the forehead and works its way cresting in intensity over the top and sides of my head, then down the neck, rolling into my shoulders in anesthetizing sensation. I can feel the pressure. At first, I panicked; tried to stop it, but I couldn't. So, I tried to learn to dance with it. But I suck at dancing. On a good day, the rhythm is smooth, though out of step in places. On a bad day, the beat is off—stumbling with two left cerebral feet over time, place, and person.

But I now have a repertoire of banter always at the ready on sports, politics, and religion for those who want to go deep. It's a defense mechanism, while I try to find my bearings. I play a game with myself, upping the stakes every day—how long can I pull this off without someone noticing? There are times when the conversation drifts to a disparate subject with no grounding, and a friend or colleague will ask politely, "You with us?" And there have been times when I have emailed a client a newspaper piece on a story pitch, carefully checking the story for date and subject matter, only to find out later that the clip was several years old and had nothing to do with the story at hand. I lost a $5,000 monthly retainer that way. I don't blame the client; I blame myself. I blame the disease.

Such mental collapses are motivation to dig deeper into the cognitive reserve, knowing in the moment that I can't go to the tank forever. The process of fighting off symptoms is exhausting, and yet exhilarating when one succeeds. It is a forceful fight for clarity, one that I win more than I lose now. For me, it's akin to the olfactory phenomenon displayed in Atlantic herring, alewives, as they make their annual migration at the strike of spring—just down the street through the ancient Brewster Herring Run, thousands of them fighting, like salmon, against a flush of water, as the alewives rush in gut instinct up the slick, steep water stone ladders of the run from Cape Cod Bay to the Upper Mill Pond to spawn in fresh water kettle ponds where they were born. The fish repeatedly are flushed back by cascading water, hitting fish heads on rocks, yet instinctively climb the ladder again.

Cognitive reserve in primal nature! Late mentor John Hay wrote about the Brewster marvel in his inspiring book, *The Run*, connecting dots to the survival instinct in all of us. "The fish kept moving up," he observed. "I watched the swinging back and forth with the current, great-eyed, sinewy, probing, weaving, their dorsal fins cutting the surface, their ventral fins fanning, their tails flipping and sculling. In the thick, interbalanced crowd there would suddenly be a scattered dashing, coming up as quickly as cat's-paws flicking the summer seas. They have moved by 'reflex' rather than conscious thought."

Conscious thought is survival; loss of reason is demise. In Alzheimer's, one fights against the drifts, those vacant staring moments when the mind floats, and you can't control it. And then there are the visual misperceptions—the polite phrase for hallucinations. They started several years ago. One night watching ESPN Sports Center, after nothing stronger than coffee with milk, I noticed some insect-like creatures, with stringy, hairy legs crawling along the top of the ceiling toward me. It wasn't the sports scores. I watched in horror as they inched closer. It was like the bar scene in *Star Wars*; they crept from wall to wall, then began to float toward me in packs. I remembered my mother telling me about them. So, I brushed them away. They vanished, though I was in a cold sweat. They kept returning at different times of day, about once every few weeks. They still come. Sometimes in packs, sometimes alone, often appearing as a spider or some other distorted vision. Sometimes they come in an army, like the time I was in Phoenix two years ago at the house of my old friend, Ray Artigue, a communications analyst and former vice president with the Phoenix Suns. I was awake in a guest room at about 8 am, and a phalanx of the imagined approached me. I swiped at them; they disappeared.

The hallucinations don't frighten me any more; Mom taught me that they will come, and they will go. An artist herself, she often counseled about fear: turn the tapestry over. Don't look at the threads beneath it, just look at the art, and don't be afraid to move on.

So I do, and keep evoking an anecdote of the great Protestant reformer Martin Luther, a man of incredible faith, who in the 1500s was frequently terrorized by his personal demons. One morning, as the anecdote goes, Luther awoke to Satan in full horror sitting at the bottom of his bed. Luther, at first, was terrified, then realized he had the faith to press on.

"Oh, it's just you again," he said to the apparition.

Then turned over and went back to sleep, like a rock.

****

Rocks have always held my attention, ever since I was a kid vacationing on Cape Cod. Leaving the Cape at the end of summer was always a sad experience for me. I can remember the empty feelings as I filled my duffel bag—the sneakers with the holes in the tips, my jeans with sand in the pockets, a surfing jam bleached by the sun, my wrinkled baseball cap—and carted it out to the station wagon. It always seemed to rain that day.

About a half hour before the family was ready to leave, all ten of us, I would take one final walk from the cottage off

Herring Brook Road in Eastham to nearby Thumpertown Beach on Cape Cod Bay. Along the way, I'd relive the summer—days fishing on Salt Pond, the time we hiked to the old Coast Guard station, the bicycle rides along the back roads to Orleans, the soothing pounding of the ocean, the sweet smell of beach plums. Each memory was precious as time was slipping away.

When I reached the bluffs of the beach, I paused for one last look with the hope that I could freeze the moment in my mind. I then walked down the wooden steps to the beach—each of the 32 planks creaking from summer wear and tear; the gray paint peeling back; many of the nails rusted from the sea air. I could see the charred remains of Labor Day campfires that had blazed the night before. Once on the beach, I ceremoniously walked, as I did each year, to the surf.

There is something about a Cape Cod summer that no other summer place can match: The sky is brighter, the sun more radiant, the sand softer, the air more pure, the mood more peaceful. Like many before me, I sought some tangible connection to this fragile, narrow sliver of land—something, a part of me, which I could leave behind. And so, each year at this time, I would walk the beach looking for a special rock, a memory to file deep within. It had to be perfect in every detail—symmetric, polished, and about the size of my fist. It had to have just the right feel. It had to feel a part of me.

I usually picked up about three-dozen rocks until I found the right one—my selected memory of that Cape Cod summer. The rejects were tossed into the bay for more polishing. I then walked back to the staircase and buried my treasure about 12 inches from the foot of the stairs.

All winter long in New York, I'd think of my rock; the summer memories it conjured helped me through the dreary days.

Then, each summer when we returned to the Cape, the first thing I'd do, after unpacking the duffel bag, was to race to the beach to retrieve the rock. I always found it, of course. I had convinced myself—and tried to persuade my mother—that any rock of similar size was the one I had stored. I collected these rocks in the back yard of the cottage we always rented, walking over them barefoot, at times, like a cobblestone path to a paradise.

I'd like to think they're still there.

9

AMERICAN PIE

WESTCHESTER COUNTY WAS AMERICAN PIE IN THE '60S. You could drink whiskey in Rye when I was young. Growing up here, just four exits up Route 95 from the Bronx, yet time zones away in culture, one could order the best brand of Bushmills on an 18th birthday. I did, and paid the price at the Five Points on Midland Avenue, now Kelly's Sea Level bar, owned today by a childhood buddy, Jerry Maguire, and his family—hardly the alter ego of Tom Cruise.

By all measure, Rye is more than a bar stop. It's a storied place on Long Island Sound at the mouth of New York Harbor, the locus of Rye Beach and Playland where movies scenes from *Fatal Attraction* with Glen Close and *Big* with Tom Hanks were filmed. I will always remember the scene in *Big* with Zoltar the Magnificent, the fortune telling machine that transported a young Hanks, the character of Josh Baskin, from childhood to adulthood and back. Where is Zoltar when I need him?

Rye is a place of long-term memories for me, a shoring up of a past that can never be forgotten—memories that offer great solace at tangents of a change in life. In Alzheimer's, brain cells in charge of short-term memory are losing the war. But long-term memory is still safely tucked away in a relatively peaceful neighborhood. Those memories are like a loyal, trustworthy friend, an ally to spend time with, at least for now. The significance and yet illusiveness of memory for those with Alzheimer's is edifying. We all need memories; they define us. Saul Bellow, the Pulitzer and Nobel Prize winner, once observed, "They keep the wolf of insignificance from the door."

Rye, in so many ways, defines my mother and me, and a legion of ethnic transplants, in its simplicity, idealism, and in the everyday ordinary that delineated a time and space, silhouetted by the demographics of a generation—long-term memories to hold tight. Rye was everyone's town. In the 1950s and '60s, it was a Norman Rockwell community from central casting, a mix of Stockbridge and *Mayberry R.F.D.*—bleached, white picket fences, flannel shirts and faded jeans, Oxford button downs from the Prep Shop on Purchase Street, and some Sax Fifth Avenue suits for the city folk.

I've never left my childhood; I exist there today, to every extent possible, moments frozen in time of great joy, peace, security, immaturity, and potty talk at times. On some days, it's the only peace I know. Alzheimer's brings one home to long-term memory—in my case, to a time when doctors made house calls, nuns wore black sweaty wool 19th century habits, baseball was king, and a McDonald's hamburger, fries, and a Coke cost just 25 cents. The memories keep me whole, and serve to stitch a patchwork quilt of experiences that leave indelible images of a life that cannot be forgotten.

Rye was the quintessence of *American Pie.* The Big Bopper,

Buddy Holly, and Ritchie Valens were icons in my town, and the night a single engine Beechcraft Bonanza, model 35, serial #D-1019, wing number N3794N, crashed in a Clear Lake, Iowa cornfield on February 3, 1959 was the day the music died here. I was in the third grade when the plane went down, and even Sister Timothy, a plump, stern, but benevolent Sister of Charity, took note of the loss. We called her the "Big Bopper."

The day the music died was the first communal tragedy Boomers experienced, a shared loss of innocence to be followed in four years by the assassination of John F. Kennedy, and three decades later by the death of Mickey Mantle, the "last boy." No doubt, the Father, Son, and Holy Ghost of a generation took the last train to the coast. But we Baby Boomers survived, a bit tougher, more cerebral, and always idealistic. Perhaps we should have seen a flood of disasters and dementias coming, like the rise of high tide on a foggy Long Island Sound. But instead, we chose to clip priceless Joe DiMaggio, Mickey Mantle, Roger Maris, and Willie Mays baseball cards with wooden clothespins to the spokes of our bicycles to mimic the roar of a motorcycle. Made us feel childishly reckless. In street value today, we shredded the collective investment of college tuitions and retirement. And we think we're so smart.

Rye—a place where George Washington slept, Ogden Nash and Amelia Earhart lived, and once the seaside retreat of the Manhattan elite—was inhabited decades ago by ethnic, first-generation working stiffs. Today, some of the wealthiest, most successful in the nation live here. But to me, Rye simply is home, a place to remember, a patchwork quilt of hometowns across the country. Everyone needs a memory of home, real or imagined; mine is more real than imagined. Innocence, as it was elsewhere, was the coin of Rye in the '50s and '60s—a town where first-, second-, and third-generation Irish and Italian Americans bonded with Jews, connecting on ball fields and sandlots here and in neighboring Port Chester. Young Italians from "the Port," as we called it in button-down Rye, often cruised Milton Road on Friday nights, beating the shit out of us Irish guys in madras shorts, pink shirts, and deck shoes. I don't blame them now. I grew up with an ethnic mix in Rye and Port Chester, regular guys like Tommy Casey, Jimmy Fitzpatrick, Vinny Dempsey, Jimmy Dianni, Billy St. John, Tony Keating, Ritchie O'Connell, Al Wilson, Brian Keefe, Chuck Drago, Dino Garr, Carlo Castallano, Rocco LaFaro, Tancredi Abnavoli, Dante Salvate, Ronald Carducci, Ritchie Breese, Micky DiCarlo, and yes, Ricky Blank, one of the most gifted Jewish shortstops I've ever known.

Many of us played organized baseball on the same teams together after we realized that an infield rundown was more fun than a slap down—later communally on a hold-your-breath, mix-and-match Rye/Port Chester All-Star Team that twice won the New York State Senior Babe Ruth League Championship with two trips to the Senior Babe Ruth League World Series regional tournament—a non sequitur of young jocks if there ever was one. In time, we all became best of friends. Six of our starters signed major league contracts. I was among those who didn't, but as a catcher, faithfully wore the tools of ignorance, first presented in the third grade at a Pony League practice.

Rye was a melting pot, boiled to perfection by the nuns. The town was predominately WASP—a hornet's nest, in fact, with three Presbyterian churches and one Catholic church, as well as a synagogue. But you could have fooled us fraternal Catholics, who reproduced like rabbits. We were tokens, often looked down upon in social circles, at the country clubs, and in line for groceries at the A&P, but we thought we owned the damn place. And in spirit, we did.

At Resurrection Grammar School, sandwiched between Milton Road and the Boston Post Road, and in the shadows of the Church of the Resurrection, a Gothic stone cathedral, one hardly messed with the nuns whose names sounded like the guest list of 1ˢᵗ century saints in Jerusalem. Sisters Timothy, Syra, Turibius, Aloysius, Monica, and Joseph, along with a convent full of accomplices had your back, your front, your top, and your bottom. But don't screw with them. You moved only on command. Our parents exceedingly impressed this dictum on us. It seems so wildly anachronistic, looking back. My parents, as most of the day, sung in this choir of didactic discipline. Church was second to family, first at times. Discipline was the order of the day. My dad, with oak-like roots in County Clare, was the first-born son of Edmund and Helen (Clancy) O'Brien; He was raised with his brother Larry by his mother's sister, Annette, and her husband, Bob O'Dell (who never missed one of my baseball games), on gritty Sedgwick Avenue in the Bronx in the shadows of the "House that Ruth Built," where he played his sandlot baseball on a diamond whose pitcher's mound today is second base in the new Yankee Stadium. His parents died of tuberculosis, the quick consumption, when he was a young boy.

My father was schooled at St. Nicholas of Tolentine and Fordham University, was one of the youngest Naval LST captains in World War II. A cerebral type, he read four newspapers a day in his professional years for a balance of news and opinion: *The New York Times, Wall Street Journal, New York Daily News,* and the *New York Post.*

He was a "layman reader" at Resurrection, one of the first ever in the church when Mass in 1969, at the decree of Pope Paul VI, was transformed from Latin to the vernacular. When Dad, an everlasting Yankee fan, was named to head up this new order of laymen, we in the family thought of him as Moses with hair dye. In a papal order from Rome, *"Ad Déum qui laetíficat juventútem méam,"* was rendered "to God who giveth joy to my youth." Not the same ring of high-church elegance to it, and besides, the English translation extended the length of a Mass. One could always burble through the Latin: *Mea Culpa, Mea Culpa, Mea Maxima Culpa!* Our pastor, Monsignor John D.

McGowan, an arthritic pastor in his 80s, still holds the record for saying Mass from start to finish in 12 minutes, including the homily. As a plebe altar boy, I served Mass that day and clocked him, as fellow altar boys looked on with pride. The aging McGowan genuflected as quickly as a wideout making a cut for the end zone.

I couldn't wait to race home to tell my mother, a beautiful woman, barely five-feet tall and a hundred pounds with platinum blond hair. "A lean horse for a long race," my dad would always say. Mom was all about the church and was impressed with such records. Raised in the shadows of the American Museum of Natural History and Hayden Planetarium in New York, she played hopscotch on the sidewalk at a time when milk was delivered in a horse-drawn carriage. Mom was educated at a French convent school and later at the College of New Rochelle in the Ursuline tradition, the first Catholic college for women in New York. Few women in the day went to college; most stayed home to have babies. A teacher later in life, she first worked as a banker, far ahead of a long awaited shattering of the glass ceiling for women, and then she became a devoted mother, deeply involved in Resurrection as a Cub Scout and Brownie leader. Life for us at the time was the epitome of the 1950s sitcom "Leave It to Beaver," exemplifying the idealized suburban family of the mid-20th century. My mother—God bless you, Eddie Haskell—frequently wore a lovely red dress.

Both parents, respectively, were members in good standing of the parish Mothers' and Fathers' Clubs. They also taught CCD, "The Confraternity of Christian Doctrine," established in Rome in 1562 for the purpose of giving religious education to the heathens. In later days, the nuns defined heathens as the children of Catholic parents who weren't sent to Catholic School. Faithful parishioners taught CCD on Wednesday nights; the nuns instructed the heathens on Thursdays at 1:30 pm, as if caring for lepers. We were dismissed early on those days. Officially, it was called "Released Time," and we were told to clear the playground as quickly as possible. The collective body language suggested that we scatter swiftly from the heathens and Huns. *Run home to the bosom of your mothers,* the nuns admonished us!

And God help us, Jesus, if we ever looked at a Protestant! We were warned never to gape at the spiral of the nearby Gothic Rye Presbyterian Church, designed in the 1860s by Richard Upjohn, the renowned church architect who built Trinity Church on Wall Street. If we even stared at this magnificent edifice, we feared, it would be akin to looking back at Sodom. We'd be turned to pillars of salt.

The mile walk from pastoral Brookdale Place to Resurrection was problematic for me. I had to pass the towers of Babel, careful not to glance up, just look down at my scuffed Buster Browns. My sisters, brothers, and I walked to school every day—the girls were dressed in the uniform of plaid skirts, white blouses, blue jackets, and black patent leather shoes; the boys were required to wear a white-collared dress shirt with a blue tie, gray flannel pants, a blue blazer, and dark socks; we all looked like Encyclopedia Britannica salesmen. The only exception to the socks rule was gym day. On gym days, guys wore white socks with running shorts underneath their trousers for a quick change in the basement for a stinging game of dodgeball or stickball in the playground. To this day, one can detect someone who was educated in the metropolitan New York Catholic school system; they will often quip at work to a friend or colleague wearing white socks: "Got gym today?"

Once at school, regardless of the temperature, five below or pushing 90, we gathered in the playground behind the red brick schoolhouse before the start of class. We were sorted in grades by cracks in the pavement. It was a blueprint to avoid chaos, the equivalent today of those invisible electronic dog fences. If you crossed the line, you'd be zapped by the nuns, unless you were queued up at the convent steps to carry the bags—the nuns' briefcases, not the old battle-axes themselves. "Brown nosers" like me waited as hungry puppy dogs outside the convent to carry a black bag; I often wondered later if they contained the nuclear code in case Khrushchev stepped out of line. At the back door of the school about 200 feet away, the exchange was made: a pat on the head, a passing of the bag, a return to the playground. We then waited within our assigned cracks, engaged in kickball, punchball, flipping cards, or just yapping. Minutes later with great thunder, an oversized glass window in the principal's office opened—an ancient kind that moved on string cords, not tracks, and made a noise like the trumpeting of angels in the Book of Revelations. The hairy, muscular arm of the Mother Superior then reached out with a cowbell the size of a boxcar. She flushed three times:

DA-DING, DA-DING, DA-DING.

The first ding ordered us to stop in motion. Instantly. Didn't matter if you were in the air, mid-sentence, or taking a pee in the hedges: you held the position. The second ding was a call to line up in silence like prisoners of war; the third ding heralded our entrance to the cellblock, err, school. All in stillness, mind you, looking straight ahead. The nuns excoriated the boys that there was to be no staring down at the shiny patent leather shoes of coeds to see their undergarments in reflection. Of course, none of us had ever thought that was possible, but what a great freakin' idea.

In class, we had 30 to 40 kids packed to a room, and hardly anyone stepped out of line. There were always exceptions. The nuns, with cold stares, would burn your retinas with a force that would frost a lawn. In the first grade, Sister Syra took no prisoners. If you were out of line, you were hung out to dry in the "clothes cupboard." Literally. In those days, the blue blazers had collar loops made of tin, and if you acted out, Sister Syra hung you on a cupboard hook like a piece of meat until your mom claimed you at the end of school, or if you happened to have a more modern blazer, the ones with a cloth loop, you were relegated to a crouch position under her desk. The discipline, while clearly over the top and flirting with abuse, had a stinging influence on me. I was afraid to go to class and skipped school one day in the first grade, hiding out in a side altar of church, one designated for Our Lady of Perpetual Help. The nuns, realizing I was AWOL went nuts. My mom was called, and the boy hunt was on. Mom ultimately determined that I was probably hiding in a pew. In short order, I was returned to class.

Second grade with amicable Sister Monica was a slide, but third grade and beyond was a call to arms. Sister Timothy would slap you silly in the mind; Sister Anthony in the fourth grade sported a moustache, and I thought I saw her once on a black-and-white television heavyweight wrestling match against champion Bruno Sammartino from Abruzzi, Italy; and Sister Joseph in the eighth grade, a long, thin women who looked remarkably like the Wicked Witch of the East, could cut right to the heart!

"I'll get you, my little pretties, and your little dogs, too!"

I still recoil at the thought of what seemed like a long, bony index finger, the length of a tractor trailer in my young imagination, reaching down a row of desks to pluck by the chin an insubordinate and carry them, on the sheer strength of hand ligaments, all the way to the front of the class for a holy thrashing, then a trip to the principal's office for yet another ceremonial kick in the ass.

Our classroom was a cattle call with the likes of incorrigible Jimmy Dianni, my alter ego in some ways, a guy who rose later in life to the position of lieutenant and chief fire inspector in the Rye Fire Department.

Dianni's foil was a classically awkward, blameless kid of the day; let's call him Liam Kelley, to protect the innocent. Kelley likely now heads up a Fortune 500 company, but Mom always felt sorry for him; she had a heart for the muddled and affronted. We've all had them in class, and many of us will do hard time in Purgatory for not coming to their relief. But as Divine or dumb luck would have it, the nuns always found a way to fuse the two—Dianni and Kelley, repelling magnets. I looked on as a voyeur just for the mere fascination of it.

Serendipity, possibly, but it all started in the fourth grade when Dianni, a freckled-faced, slightly chubby boy, hurled, for some enigmatic reason, his tattered brown book bag, the kind with silver metal corners at the bottom, into a crowded playground. Perhaps he was just mad at his mother. But who did it hit right in the squash? Kelley! Was it by design? Maybe just dumb freakin' luck? But, game on!

****

Halloween, no doubt, was in the air late on a Friday afternoon in October in the early 1960s. Dead, fallen oak leafs were swept by a coastal wind across the asphalt parking lot at Resurrection, like screaming pucks at a hockey practice, as the nuns herded us from the bulky red brick school building to Resurrection Church for weekly hymn practice for the obligatory 10 am Sunday Mass, which students and families were all expected to attend; the nuns took names at the church door. At this particular Friday practice, Sister Aloysius was orchestrating like Leonard Bernstein—spine upright, arms pumping in baton-like fashion, thick white-matted hair beneath her black bonnet. We filed into the church like lambs to a slaughter; no one was allowed to speak; we were entering "Oz" after all. We were warned: Nobody talks to the Wizard. God has the whole world in his hands, and frankly, there's no room for you. So, buck up, just sit in silence, pray the Rosary, hope you're not struck by lightning, and listen up for further orders. I got it, but Jimmy missed it.

For some delightful reason, maybe the sheer pleasure of it, the nuns positioned Dianni in a pew next to Kelley, who sat unaffected up against a granite pillar that rose from the floor to the roof of the church that seemed to us the height of the Empire State Building. On this particular Friday, I was sitting to the left of Dianni; Kelley was to the right of him, plumb against a cold stone pillar with enough room between the pew and pillar for a small pumpkin. We were rehearsing the hymn *Army of God* in full, uplifted voice:

> *And I hear the sound of the coming rain,*
> *As we sing the praise to the Great I Am*
> *And the sick are healed, and the dead will rise*
> *And your church is the army that was prophesied*

As the chorus reached its holy peak, and the Lord's grace was raining down on us, we could hear a piercing cry from the back of the church.

"Get my head out! Get my head out!"

Kelley had dropped his hymnal between the pew and the pillar, and Dianni obliged on cue by wedging Kelley's head between them.

"Get my head out!" Kelley yelled in a voice that overpowered the saints.

"Dianni, you fuck, get my head out!"

The sisters were apoplectic. They raced to the back of the church as if someone had just burned down a convent full of nuns. At the scene of the crime, a decision was made to call in church sexton, John Quinn—a gnarly man with a brogue as thick as Guinness and looking a bit like Bilbo Baggins in *Lord of the Rings*. He was asked to pry the swelled head loose. With the sturdy hands of an apostle rebuking the devil himself, Quinn safely extracted the head intact.

"It's free, it's free!" he declared, having snatched Kelley's head from what all had feared were the jaws of death.

With baton still in hand, and looking as if she had just witnessed a vomit scene from *The Exorcist*, Sister Aloysius tersely dismissed hymn practice. "I think we've sung enough today!" she said, the pleats of her habit swaying with a shake of her knees.

The imbroglio ensued, and I looked on in awe of Jimmy, yet with a guilt of Jesuit proportions, but I knew that Kelley would have his day. Witnessing the conflict refined me in calculation of character, moments in long-term memory that I can never forget. It is reassuring for me.

Months later, with 38 students sandwiched in math class, authoritarian Sister Joseph ended the session with a repressive homework assignment from our *Progress In Arithmetic* textbook. The room groaned as if crushed by a school bus. Dianni, sitting again next to Kelley, goaded him to protest, and Sister Joseph became enraged at the class defiance.

"Add to your assignment," she ordered, "the worksheet at the end of chapter two!" she ordered.

The moans continued with Kelley leading the charge.

"And just for that, copy all the times tables in the back of the book, three times!" Sister Joseph declared, as if challenged by the underworld.

The wailing subsided, although some laments could still be heard. Dianni prodded Kelley again for a response. Kelley was waiting to pounce.

"Fine," Sister Joseph screamed, the veins in her neck popping, that long index finger poised. "We're gonna have a test tomorrow on the first four chapters!"

There was a frightening silence. Sister Joseph had prevailed.

Not so quick. Dianni looked at Kelley, Kelley looked at Dianni, and then Kelley cried out, *"Ah shit!"*

The words echoed throughout the classroom. Sinewy Sister Joseph sprinted to the back of the room and pounced like a linebacker. What was left of Kelley seconds later was sent to the principal's office.

But God is good, justice is certain, and in Dublin, one never gets mad, right? Kelley retaliated in time.

****

A rite of passage at Resurrection in the seventh grade was the day students moved up from writing in lead pencil to fountain pen, filled to the brim of the cartridge with blue India ink. A successor of the dip-pen that Ben Franklin once used to sign the Declaration of Independence, the fountain pen had a stainless steel or gold nib that washed a wave of ink onto a page. You had to write fast, or the ink flooded; a practical reality that may have taught us Baby Boomers to think quicker when writing.

A bottle of precious blue India ink rested on the oak eraser ledge below the blackboard, and one approached the ledge for refilling the fountain pen with all the reverence of standing before the Holy Grail. The nuns had taught us that it was a mystical privilege to write in blue ink. One day in the seventh grade, I saw Kelley in line for ink; he had the look of a gunman, as the rest of the class sat passively in their seats, blue jackets off, white shirts exposed. Kelley filled the cartridge slowly and deliberately, getting every ounce possible into the reservoir. He turned with intent, walked down the middle aisle toward Dianni's desk, his eyes affixed to the back of the room so as not to draw attention. Passing Dianni, still in stride, he waved his pen in a fierce jerky motion in front of Dianni's new clean white shirt, the one his mother had warned him not to soil. In an instant, a large "Z," the size of the Mark of Zorro, was indelibly imprinted on Dianni's shirt. Kelley, in the role of the swashbuckling Don Diego de la Vega, a.k.a. Zorro, had left his mark on Dianni, now the dupe, and relegated to the role of Sergeant Demetrio López García.

Nobody messes with Zorro. Class dismissed.

Seasoned altar boys, Jimmy (in his makeshift pinstripe shirt) and I immediately fled for the sanctuary of the church—not for the confessional, but to light up incense in a closet of a room off the sanctuary. The Catholic Church interprets the burning of incense as a symbol of the Prayer of the Faithful, rising to Heaven, a purification process. The incense is burned in a metal container called a thurible, to be dispensed in three ritual swings for the Trinity. The imagery is recorded in Psalm 141:2, "Let my prayer be directed as incense in thy sight: the lifting up of my hands, as evening sacrifice."

But Jimmy and I weren't there for the prayer. We just liked the smell of the stuff. Besides, as captain of the school safety patrol and altar boy Master of Ceremonies, a position in the church pecking order akin to Michael the Archangel, I had access to the room. Keys to the Kingdom. It pleased my mother; she was also proud of the way we held sway with the nuns at Mass. Jimmy taught me to hold the gold-plated altar communion plate just above the Adam's apple of nuns queued up for communion. When the sisters lined up, we would press the plate gently against their throats, just to let them know we were there. A presence almost as good as a supernatural power.

Jimmy always has been a presence with me. Fifty years later, when he learned that I had been diagnosed with Alzheimer's, he called to express his love and support; he promised me that he wasn't going to treat me any differently. It was music to my ears. He ended the conversation with a play on Alzheimer's: "Remember, buddy, you still owe me a hundred bucks!" I've passed the exchange along to other friends, who have responded in kind, "You owe me a hundred bucks, too! And don't forget it."

Bada-bing, bada-boom.

****

The boom came in October 1962 with the Cuban missile crisis of the Cold War, a 13-day war of words between the U.S., the Soviet Union, and its ally Cuba—a Russian roulette among titans of the day—Soviet Premier Nikita Khrushchev, Cuban Prime Minister Fidel Castro, and John F. Kennedy. No one was ready to blink.

Two months earlier, after unsuccessful covert U.S. operations to overthrow Castro through a failed Bay of Pigs invasion and Operation Mongoose, the Cubans and Soviets secretly began constructing medium-range and intermediate-range ballistic nuclear missile bases with the ability to strike most of the continental U.S. Photo reconnaissance captured proof. It is generally regarded as the moment the world came closest to nuclear holocaust. After rejecting tactics of attacking Cuba by air and sea, the Kennedy brain trust opted for a naval blockade of Cuba—no Soviet ship would be allowed to enter Cuban waters. In a letter to Kennedy, Khrushchev called the blockage "an act of aggression, propelling humankind into the abyss of a world nuclear-missile war."

"Ah, shit!" as Kelley would say.

On October 25, 1962, the Soviet ships were steaming just off Cuba, and the U.S. was not standing down. We were on the edge of extinction, we thought. The nuns were abuzz with images of Armageddon, and tuned-in transistor AM radios throughout Resurrection for the holy unwashed to hear. Last call for us, and no one had passed the height line yet at the Five Points. After wet-your-pants radio reports and a mock class exercise of duck and cover under our desks in the event of a nuclear attack (as if to vaporize us in a position of kissing our asses goodbye), the bell rang to end school, and we all spilled out of the building like flushing tap water, down the second floor stairs, to the first floor, heading to the back door. Billy St. John and I then hung a quick right to the basement.

"Where are you guys going?" cautioned Tony Keating, a life-long friend, who walked home with us every day. "Keats, we're going to the basement to get ready for the boys' basketball team tryouts," replied Billy.

Few seventh graders had ever made the eighth-grade team, and Billy and I were on the precipice of greatness, hoping Coach Pete McHugh would tap us.

Keating stopped us in our tracks. "Where do you want to be when the bomb drops? On the basketball court with Mr.

McHugh, or home with your parents where you belong?"

The logic was unassailable. And so, like lemmings, we followed Keating down Milton Road to safe haven. When I got home, I hugged my mom, and then went to my room to pray.

"Dear God, not now, please not now!"

Prayers were answered. The next day, no bomb. Kennedy and Khrushchev had agreed in back-channel negotiations that the Soviets would dismantle offensive weapons in Cuba, and the U.S., in return, would agree not to invade Cuba and dismantle missiles in Turkey and Italy. Still, Billy and I were cut from the eighth-grade team for missing practice and racing home to pray. A small price, I suppose, for saving the world.

Prayer was always a part of the daily routine at Resurrection, drilled into our thick "cabezas" through all the smoke and mirrors of *Mad Magazine* and *Playboy* centerfolds. Every May, we had special devotions to the Blessed Virgin Mary, honoring the mother of Christ as the "Queen of May," a ritual that dated back to the 16th century. We were all schooled in the virginity of Mary, and many of us, at the direction of the priests, nuns, and our parents, wore scapulars—the Blue Scapular of the Immaculate Conception, scratchy cloth images of the Blessed Virgin that were suspended over the chest and the back by thin twine. While often causing a rash, the scapular came with a sacred promise, known as the Sabbatine Privilege, that the Blessed Virgin, through special intercession on the Saturday after the death of a devotee, would personally liberate and deliver the soul from Limbo.

I was all over that.

On May Day, the nuns instructed us to write private letters to the Blessed Virgin, our personal prayer requests, nothing to be held back. It was to be a solemn exercise. We were then assembled, as if awaiting the Rapture, at the rear of the parking lot behind the church, in front of a tall granite statue of the Blessed Virgin. At the base of the statue was a large wire bin into which we tossed our prayers to Mary. Then, Sexton Quinn, on orders, lit the prayers on fire, and we all watched our words drift up to Heaven in the smoke. I could see them.

Still can.

Each year, I had the same prayer: that my mom and dad would live forever.

10

Forget-Me-Nots

In the spring on Brookdale Place, the forget-me-nots bloomed like a botanical garden, a sea of soothing pastels that kindle the memory. The Greeks called the flower Myosotis, translated "mouse's ear," an allusion to the shape of its leaf. Who could ever forget a patch of ensuring Forget-Me-Nots, delicate five-lobed blue, pink or white flowers with yellow centers? German folklore says the Almighty once overlooked the petite plant in naming all the other flowers. Legend suggests that one of the tiny lobes cried out, "Forget-me-not, Oh Lord." To which God replied, "That shall be your name."

Often in life, we remember the diminutive. Henry David Thoreau wrote of Forget-Me-Nots, "It is the more beautiful for being small and unpretending; even flowers must be modest."

I grew up in a modest neighborhood where memories last

forever. Forever is a long time, yet in a long-term memory, it's a place of persistent peace, a steadfast mooring when the swift high tides of life pull one to treacherous waters where memory implores the brain: forget me not.

****

It took forever in Rye for our stickball games to end on Brookdale Place. Used to drive my mother nuts, as she tried diligently to prepare dinner in two shifts for ten. Most of the time was taken up trying to find the errant ball in Phil Clancy's shrubs or Mr. Androtti's ivy, or secure another broom handle for a bat when we had exhausted our stash. I used to sneak broom handles out of the rectory at Resurrection Church, telling Bridie, the matronly Irish woman who cared for the priests, that I needed another broom to sweep the sidewalks for Monsignor McGowan.

Bridie was a tough Gaelic doyenne; it was difficult to discern her age from the deep crevices in her face and her youthful voice. She was always accommodating, but she intuitively knew that I was up to something, yet seemed to enjoy the repartee. After securing another boom, I always tried to do something helpful on my way out of the rectory, like putting a plate away in the kitchen or a glass back on another shelf, usually a spot where Bridie had just baked a stack of chocolate chip cookies.

"Anything else I can do for you?" I would ask with a handful of plunder in one palm, the prospective stickball bat in the other.

"Yeah," she always replied, "stick that broom up your ass and sweep the floor!"

When Bridie's stock ran out, we looked to Jim O'Rourke, the guy from Killarney that looked two decades beyond his age; the priests had hired him to cut the lawn. Jim loved to drink, and usually began about 10 am, walking down to McGuire's Market, owned by Jerry's dad, for a morning Bud, while most in the store were looking for the cream. By noon, O'Rourke was usually sleeping it off in the janitor's room; so we'd sneak in and steal a broom. He lost a lot of brooms on the job.

But we never lost the bases on Brookdale Place. We didn't need to take them home at night. The field was the street, long and narrow like the fairways at St. Andrew's. First base was the birch tree on the curb lip in front of Pappy Langeloh's house; second base was the large, sweeping oak in front of Lou Kelly's home; and third base was the blunt edge of Ronnie Buckie's driveway. Home plate was chalked in the middle of the street, batter's box and all.

As often as we could, we'd have Hungarian born Zena Kelly, Lou's trophy wife, throw out the first ball for special effects. She was Zsa Zsa Gabor incarnate to us kids. She had some big *casabas*, knew it, and always obliged us. Al Wilson frequently dropped the ball when handing it to her for the opening toss. I don't know if he was just nervous like Hermie in the *Summer of '42*, or he was just looking for Zena to pick it up. Al was no fool.

Mom often watched from the kitchen window, her fixed position over time, as she gazed out, taking it all in, sorting out what it all meant or what she thought it to be, as she often talked to herself or to an imaginary friend. The conversations continued. Over the years, the neighborhood stickball players came and went, depending on age. If you could swing a bat and stood taller than a tricycle, you could play.

The regulars included my brothers Paul, Tim, and Andy; my tomboy sister, Lauren, a pretty good hitter, also played from time to time. My sister, Maureen, a "Hot Lips" Houlihan-type, frequently watched from the sidewalk, as did sisters Justine and Bernadette from their scooters.

Stickball, a variation of a Northeast inner city game invented in the 1750s, takes ample coordination, but if you hit the sweet spot of the broom handle, you could drive the pink Spalding high-bounce ball, the Spaldeen, almost to Monument Park in Yankee Stadium. The crowd always cheered as the ball lifted, like a Project Mercury rocket, above the canopy of trees—

prompted by a din from deep inside the throat of the slugger, as he mimicked the roar of a standing ovation, pushing gusts of air up the esophagus, then instinctively limping into a Mickey Mantle trot, aping the weak knees of "The Mick," head cocked to the left for balance.

"Holy cow! Did you see that?" we mocked in our best Phil Rizzuto.

We commonly ran out of digits counting the scores. Games were often called on account of the bell, not a lost ball, weather or darkness, but the bell.

We all lived by bells; I often felt like a cow. On the back porch at 25 Brookdale, Mom would ring a cowbell the size of a grapefruit with a long cord that my dad had hung from the porch ceiling. The knell was a summons for all the O'Briens, no exceptions, to head home. Game over!

Da-ding, Da-ding, Da-ding!

The clangor was a directive for the other kids to go home as well, a dictate from my mother that neighborhood parents relied on to gather their flocks. Brookdale Place was an extended family. Mom was the bell ringer, the arm of authority on a dead-end street with a tidal brook at the end that meandered to Long Island Sound. We never had to worry about speeding cars, other than some of the relatives after too many whiskey sours over the holidays. Brookdale parents watched out for every kid. We had group cookouts, block parties, and in the summer time, the neighborhood kids roamed freely through back yards playing flashlight tag or catching fireflies. Bernadette Burgess, who lived across the street, had the best swarm of fireflies.

There were few organized sports in those days; pickup was the rule: stickball, wiffle ball, stoop ball, basketball, and of course, slow-motion tackle football in the fall and winter after Pappy Langeloh had cut down his corn stocks in the field next to us. The most fun was plowing through the snowdrifts of December on fourth down and short yardage, and giving the ball on a fullback drive to four-year olds, bloated in their puffy snowsuits like the Pillsbury Doughboy.

With the largest family on the block, my folks ruled the neighborhood. There were a lot of big Irish families in Rye then. Birth control in the Catholic Church then was anathema. Judging from the size of families in Rye the "rhythm method" of birth control was working about as well in New York as Casey Stengel's curve ball. Priests and nuns, presumably most of whom never had sex, instructed mothers of the parish to recognize the days of a fertile womb and avoid intercourse—a game plan gone with the wind after a few martinis. "I got rhythm," as the Gershwin song goes.

Then bango, bingo! The wives got pregnant again. My mother gave birth to ten children and had five miscarriages—fifteen pregnancies in all. I've always considered younger brothers, Gerard and Martin, who died in infancy, part of the family, and always will. The miscarriages will remain nameless until Heaven. Large Catholic families were *de rigueur* in the day. The Caseys had eight, the Cunninghams seven, and my godmother Eileen Clavin had sixteen. Everyone used to call her, with Mother Goose distinction, the Old Woman in the Shoe:

> *...She had so many children.*
> *She didn't know what to do.*
> *She gave them some broth.*
> *Without any bread;*
> *Then whipped them all soundly.*
> *And put them to bed.*

Not really. We never got whipped at home, nor did Eileen's kids; she was an angel of a godmother. But the thought of a thumping kept us on the straight and narrow, and it was just a train ride away. My father worked in Manhattan in the old Pan Am building above Grand Central as director of pensions, a 25-minute ride on the express New Haven line. When I or one of my brothers or sisters stepped out of line, my mom threatened to place the call, and "The Belt" would be on its way. Infractions ranged from mouthing off, to failing to do chores, to bad grades, or in Lauren's case, one of her virtuoso "drop-dead" looks. Lauren, third in the pecking order, had perfected a look of contempt with trademark Irish diplomacy—the ability to tell someone to go to hell, in a way that they looked forward to the trip. I was always impressed, but Mom was on to it.

"Wait 'til your father gets home, and you're going to get the belt!"

The threat alone was sobering.

My mom, a Donna Reed mirror image, was petite, barely five-feet tall and all of 104 pounds, but she had the will, when necessary, to inflict one badass guilt trip. Her nickname in later years was "Boomer," a moniker passed down from brother-in-law Carl, a reference to a hard-hitting Minnesota Vikings tailback named Bill "Boom Boom" Brown with a reckless, almost violent running style. Like the late '60s All-Pro tailback, Mom could bowl us over, knock us right off our feet, with the largesse of her great intellect, wisdom, and ceaseless love—good and tough, always justified and in abundant measure.

I never actually saw the belt, but envisioned it laid out on my parents' bed, stiff like a corpse in a casket. The "belt" I dreaded, was a ten-foot long, four-foot wide strip of rawhide with sharp nails poking up and a belt buckle the size of a suitcase. But worse than the belt was my mom looking me squarely in the eye, cutting deep to the back of the brain stem, and declaring, "I'm disappointed in you. I thought you could do better."

Please, I'd rather the belt. Just give me the belt. A few swings and it will be over. The sting of disappointment lingered. *Ouch!*

My relationship with my mother came full circle. Growing up as the oldest boy, early on, I received a disproportionate amount of attention from my father. I adored my dad; he was my exemplar, but I always looked to my mother for inner strength. She knew my heart and the souls of all her children. But I strayed in time, and being the "free lunch" of the family, a Prodigal Son in some ways, I disappointed her, pushing the boundaries selfishly in sophomoric ways, defiant of my parents' munificence and limited resources. Mom and I didn't have much of a relationship for a time; then we found each other in Alzheimer's. End of life has a way of doing that.

Mom was big on confession. You always had to come clean with her. Confession as a youth was a ritual in our house. On Thursdays at church, you were directed to the confessional box, sort of a spiritual "time out," for a weekly unloading of a bolus of sins, often defined as missing the mark. We sat inside a dark cubicle with a dividing wire screen and a phantom, ghostly figure behind it that had all the redemption of death row. Three Hail Marys, an Our Father, and Glory Be, and you'd be on your way, off sinning again, constantly reminded to tow the line. Praise the Lord, and pass the *Playboys!*

My parents, greatly influenced by scripture, frequently read passages to us, particularly when trying to make a point on Christmas Eve, Easter, or when the spirit moved. They gave us all strong biblical or Irish names: my brother Paul for Saul of Tarsus; Timothy and Andrew for the apostles; Gregory after the writer pope, Gregory the Great, who took office in 590 AD, although I never lived up to the name; Bernadette for the miller's daughter, born in 1844 in Lourdes, France, who asserted to have seen the Virgin Mary in a cave grotto; and so on. Sometimes, Dad would let us vote on the names of new arrivals in the family, a majority of one vote; however, we did nix my dad's choice of the name Thaddeus, a disciple and close friend of the Apostle Jude, not to be confused with Judas. Like an oversized diaper, the name was too much for an infant. My mom and the voting siblings were all in agreement on this. There was no division.

Division generally is the rule in a large family, which has become a dinosaur of our culture, a Tyrannosaurus of tradition.

Either by birth order, intent, or a shuffling of the deck, or just dumb luck, my parents divided the brood into "the older kids" and the "younger kids," a classification that would appall most child psychologists today, but one that sticks, with some of the siblings retaining their birth-order roles, as do others in Boomer families. The older kids, by my parents' declaration, were consecrated to be: Maureen, me, and Lauren; the younger kids: Justine, Paul, Bernadette, Timothy, and Andy, the baby. Ironically, the baby, now an EMC Corporation executive in Manhattan, is the big breadwinner, probably making threefold the rest of us, with the exception of brother Paul, also an EMC honcho.

The family expanded exponentially over time to the point that my folks in the summer had to rent two cottages off Thumpertown Beach Road in Eastham on the Outer Cape. A colleague at Pan Am had introduced my dad to the Cape when he was in his early 30s. The older kids were dispatched to the snug, yellow cabin, next to the gray mothership of a cottage where the younger kids were kept near my parents. Maureen, Lauren, and I will never forget the night, in the early '60s in the early morning hours, when someone tried to break in the back door next to our bedroom. Looking back, I suspect it was my dad, just trying to make sure we didn't become too independent from the family. No chance of that! We all relied on one another.

Maureen, a nurse to be, was the second mother, "Mother Superior," as we called her; Lauren took no prisoners in family disparities. I was initially relegated to lawn duties with a manual push mower, trimming the front hedge with sheers, and snow shoveling the driveway. The younger kids stepped up as we stepped away, in some instances, doing a far better job. When I stepped away to pursue the low fruit of the world, no one seemed to notice.

My parents, for the most part, were exceedingly close, fully romantic in the early years, but with the heaviness of life, they became more distant, then intimate again in the final days. They were like blueberry bushes that seem to grow better in pairs. My parents were typically competitive, too, and instilled stiff competition among us, a rule of family law that kept us lean, mean, and hungry for our grades in school, and always competing for the cleanliness of the four-floor, six-bedroom stucco home we occupied. We all had Friday cleaning chores, from the finished basement to the attic. And when it came to our "marks" in school, my folks were cutthroat, particularly with the older kids. In grammar school, if we brought home a 95 percent overall academic average on a report card, it simply wasn't enough.

"You can do better," Dad would say, holding out the prize of his affection for the highest grades.

And so we were pushed to bring home 98s and 99s, which we did, and then moved on to private Catholic high schools, most of us, where we studied logic, philosophy, and learned to translate from Latin Cicero's letters and Virgil's *Aeneid*, sometimes with the help of a black-market translator called a Trot.

The CliffsNotes of our family life read like Frank Capra's *It's a Wonderful Life*. My dad was indeed George Bailey; my mom in the role of Mary Hatch. In Rye, we had our various Uncle Billys, Ernie Bishops, and Bert the cop, even an Aunt Bee and Roger the Dellwood milkman, who delivered three times a week 12 to 14 glass bottles of milk to our house and stacked them in our refrigerator. And we were surrounded by guardian angels; Clarence Odbody, I swear, lived down the street.

****

My mother was a living angel; she loved the primary color yellow. Yellow angel rays, we were taught, represent the enlightenment that the Lord's wisdom brings to the soul. Social in every respect, my mother attended all the gatherings of the day. She met my father at a college dance in New Rochelle. He was a Fordham University student at the time and a Naval officer candidate. Dad was the rudder of the family; Mom was the mainsail, and stood out among the Greatest Generation of women of her day—wives and mothers who helped shape and define their spouses and children in diverse ways, both in what they were in life and are today in memories. These women gave selflessly in child-rearing years, then later as caregivers for their war-hero husbands, never receiving a medal for it.

And in the end, the Greatest Generation of men, independent conquerors of world evil, clung to their spouses in old age; survivors still do. This generation of women has never received the accolades it deserves.

My dad needed mollycoddling. Losing his parents to tuberculosis as a young boy, he never fully recovered from the loss. An athlete, thinker, a man of letters, and a Roosevelt Democrat, my father found comfort in excelling beyond his means with a Gaelic will to succeed and sustain his passions. He was once asked at a Fordham University oral theology exam, seated before a table of schooled clerics in the shadows of high Gothic walls that seemed to reach to the Heavens, to prove there was a God. He answered with great clarity, faith, and Jesuit logic, pointing to the world around him. And today, he has the irrefutable evidence.

Holding court with us one day on the beach, he reflected on the imperfections of life, likely quoting another academic. "Life is like a river," he intoned, "You need to study it as it goes by, then decide the right time to put your feet in the water." Dad was a man who got right to the point. He once told one of my brothers: "Don't get me wrong, Greg's a nice guy, but he's like medicine; you have to take him in small doses." Yet, Dad was loving, like my mom, in what one might call marital photosynthesis: they emitted love and life to each other.

Still they were strict, always pursuing the narrow road. At times, they lost their way; as years passed, my mom, given her Alzheimer's, more so than my dad. We began to notice over the years wholesale lapses in memory and continued engagement in conversations with people and objects that weren't real. At first, we ignored it: phones left off the hook because she couldn't figure out how to end a call; wearing shoes that didn't match; those distant, vacant stares; and, at times, an out-of-body persona, a mix of aberrant rage and adolescent fancy. Still, the distractions of a large family, all the school, sporting, and church events camouflaged her illness, as well as the routine of teaching duties at parochial Most Holy Trinity in nearby Mamaroneck and St. Gregory the Great in Harrison.

In time, the symptoms worsened, more so after my parents retired to the Outer Cape in 1998, a place of further isolation in winter, a precursor to Pluto, a venue where she went from clothes shopping at Bergdorf Goodman in Manhattan to Brown's Superette for baloney in Eastham.

Mom departed from Rye reluctantly, following my dad as she had done instinctively from the day they met. She brought with her a quilt of long-term memories to last a lifetime that was now measured in short years, not decades.

I couldn't imagine until now the isolation she must have felt.

Mom left a dead-end street for a dead end in her life. As peaceful and bucolic as the Cape was, the lights were growing dimmer.

Da-ding, Da-ding, Da-ding!

Bye-bye, Miss American Pie, on to a dead-end street.

Forget me not.

11

DEAD-END STREET

CESTARO WAY IN NORTH EASTHAM IS HARDLY A PROPER name and easy to remember for a narrow lane on Cape Cod, lined with dense patches of scrub oak and scrub pine on the fringe of the Cape Cod National Seashore, about two miles from the frothing Atlantic. It's a dead-end choice, on a dead-end street. But developer Arty Cestaro wouldn't have it any other way after he bulldozed a swath of sandy forest off School House Road in the late 1960s, sold my parents two lots for a summer house, then dug a drinking well down "sixty tree" feet.

A burly, stubby Italian with a touch of Genoa in his voice, Arty was a man for all seasons on Cape Cod, all three of them. Spring arrives for a day in June.

Since the Pilgrims first arrived in these parts, year-round survival on this narrow land has required a range of cunning and skill. Depending on the time of year, Arty—who sported a face of peppered stub—cleared lots, built homes, fished for bass and blues, and baked a cloistered family recipe of thick lasagna and crusty Italian bread to sell to the tourists—all under the banner of Cestaro.

So, why not Cestaro Way?

The street was a mirror image of Arty, as it was for my family: course, bumpy, potholed, with thin strands of oak attempting to reclaim the road. It was perfect in an old Cape Cod way, just perfect. Ours was the first house built on Cestaro Way. It was a two-bedroom cottage with an unfinished attic that served as a sleeping porch for most of the kids; we camped out on molded mattresses or in sleeping bags, some with a slight hint of urine, depending on a Friday night out. The attic had a natural alarm system for wake-up calls. On hot summer days, the sun baked the framing beams and sandy plywood floors to the point of driving a deep sweat. My dad had the house built as a family retreat and for retirement. Mom, abidingly along for the ride, enjoyed the view on Cestaro, particularly from the back deck that overlooked the dense scrub pines—a place, she often said, where she could lose herself. And ultimately did.

After a decade of summers renting a nearby Thumpertown Beach cottage complex, having a place now to call home on the Cape was like pouring Super Glue over the family. We all stuck together—sand, gravel, pine needles, sweat, and all. Mom and the siblings stayed for the summer, as was the custom for summer people, and Dad flew up weekends between vacation times. My parents were immensely proud of their Cestaro Way anchor, testament to family values they wanted to share: *Mi casa es su casa!* My father covertly, yet with benevolence, hid a spare key on a rusted nail under the back porch, then proceeded to tell Arty Cestaro, the North Eastham postmaster, everyone at Betty's Beach Box and Brown's Superette, vagrants at the laundromat, all those in line for coffee at Fleming's Donut

Shack, the fishermen at Goose Hummock in Orleans, and just about everybody he met on the Cape, Manhattan, Westchester County, and all along the way. Thank God Al Gore hadn't invented the Internet yet.

Trust was a maxim of the day. Life on the Outer Cape in the '50s, '60s, and early '70s was simple and quiet, like my mother, in a Norman Rockwell way. Creation of the Cape Cod National Seashore, signed into legislation in 1961 by John F. Kennedy, who summered in Hyannisport, saw to it that some of Henry David Thoreau's pristine vistas, 43,500 acres in all, remained undisturbed. The Cape was uncomplicated then. When Jack Kennedy, for example, stopped receiving his weekly edition of *The Cape Codder* delivered to the White House, the president phoned his good friend, Malcolm Hobbs, the paper's publisher, to inquire about his favorite local read.

"Let me check on that, Jack," Malcolm said from the newsroom.

There was a pause on the phone, while Malcolm made his way back to the subscription office.

"Hey, Jack," Malcolm replied minutes later, "your subscription has run out! Send a check, and we'll send you the paper."

Kennedy laughed, fully relishing the moment amidst world convolutions. A check was dispatched, and Kennedy never missed an issue of *The Cape Coder* again.

That simple, that direct, an exchange that wholly defined the Cape decades ago, a far different place than today. The beaches were wider, ample room for the wooden playpens, sticky from apple juice, that the fathers of large families schlepped down a steep flight of wooden steps from the top of the bluff. Surfers and surf casters on the beach were as plentiful as shorebirds; beach bonfires were the proxy of a summer night on the town. We bathed with soap and shampoo in clear freshwater kettle ponds where you could see bottom 50 feet from shore; and on Saturdays just before sunset, we all raced to the sea to watch a squadron of Navy planes from Otis Air Force Base line up in a mock carpet-bombing mission to drop live, pulsating ammunition on the "Target Ship," the 417-foot U.S.S. James Longstreet, a decommissioned World War II Liberty Ship named after a Confederate general. It had been towed to a site in Cape Cod Bay a few miles offshore. The final run of the night was greeted with applause up and down the beach, as if Ted Williams had just hit another dinger. The Longstreet, rusted to submission, now lies in a shallow grave below the surface.

My mother felt safe in Eastham. We all did. The place felt to her like Rye in the '60s. There wasn't much crime on the Outer Cape: a few fisticuffs here and there and a botched drug drop or two. Nearby, Wellfleet and Truro police cruisers in those days often marked time by playing tag with spotlights in the woods; a Wellfleet police officer once had to pedal his bike to work after receiving a DWI; selectmen fought in bars after disagreeing over town business; and the kindly Wellfleet watchman, always willing to offer a helping hand, once unwittingly assisted drug smugglers unloading bulky burlap bags of marijuana off a sailboat, named *Mischief*, moored in the harbor to a waiting truck in the parking lot for flight off-Cape. When the watchman finally discerned the nature of the cargo, he called the Wellfleet police, who came screaming down to the harbor with sirens on full alert from miles away to avoid a possible gunfight. The smugglers fled; nothing was ever found, other than an embarrassed watchman. I covered the scene as a cub reporter for *The Cape Codder*. Alec Wilkinson—a gifted writer for *The New Yorker*, a successful author, and a Wellfleet summer cop in his youth—chronicled the antics, and more, in a remarkable book: *Midnights: A Year with the Wellfleet Police*.

The Outer Cape, over the years, has always attracted its share of eccentrics, and square foot by square foot, some of the finest intellectual, artistic, and writing talent in the world, who shaped the culture of a generation. Among them, writers like Eugene

O'Neill, Tennessee Williams, Sinclair Lewis, Norman Mailer, Mary Oliver, Poet Laureate Stanley Kunitz, Arthur Schlesinger, Jr., Annie Dillard, and Marge Piercy, to name a few, along with some of the most notable artists and therapists of the last century, not to mention the sweet oysters here. It's still said that you can't find a shrink in Manhattan in August because they are all vacationing on the Cape.

Hidden deep in the Wellfleet-Truro woods, not far from the Great Outer Beach, is one of Cape Cod's best kept secrets— remnants of a summer colony that once housed some of these gifted architects, diplomats, and critical thinkers from the 1930s. These homes on stilts—designed by the brightest and most inventive modernist architects in Europe and America—were functional, yet radical; sort of floating boxes, oriented to capture views and breezes, perching lightly on the land with flat roofs that often rise to gradual pitches. The buildings are as significant to the region's built environment as any antique Cape or saltbox, all part of the allure of isolation in the Outer Cape woods, a place of intense privacy for creative inspiration and low-impact buildings that were "green" long before there was such an environmental color.

And then there was intriguing Charles Flato, a hunchbacked intellectual writer who had suffered from polio as a child, worked later as an investigator reporter for the civil liberties subcommittee of the Senate Labor Committee, served under Nelson Rockefeller in the Latin American division of the Board of Economic Warfare during World War II, lived in retirement in the Wellfleet woods, and oh, yes, was a Russian spy. Flato was outed when KGB files were opened to researchers after the Soviet Union collapsed. His codename in the Gorsky memo, written by Anatoly Gorsky, then chief of Soviet intelligence, was "Bob" and in another Verona transcript, cryptanalysis of Soviet intelligence dispatches, Flato is believed to have the codename of "Char."

I thought of him as Charlie, and he was always willing to talk. He was a good local source in my early reporting days. My mother liked him as well. Charlie and I shared a plantation of coffee beans over the years on his back deck. I just thought he was a guy with a brain and a cane.

"I couldn't think of a better place to get lost," Charlie once told me.

The isolation, stark natural beauty, and anonymity of the Outer Cape drew many—the famous, infamous, and regular people, like my folks—to dead-end streets, and held them captive here.

****

The early retirement days for my parents were blissful, but the isolation finally resonated with my mother about three weeks into her first winter here, as the reality of year-round residency on this patch of sand, jutting 60 miles into the tempestuous North Atlantic, settled in with the starkness of a whiteout in a coastal storm, a place where the major highway, Route 6, resembled a walking trail in February. It never snows on the Cape, the locals promote, and you can play golf here year-round. But grab the Dramamine and check the map. "The bared and bended arm of Cape Cod," naturalist Thoreau wrote, is where "a man can stand there and put all of America behind him." The remoteness in winter on the Outer Cape, while inspiring and cerebral, is no place for someone who is losing their place. My mother never got the memo.

Neither did the Pilgrims, who never "landed" in Plymouth in the strict definition of the term. They anchored instead off Provincetown on the Cape's tip on November 11, 1620 where William Bradford, the first Plymouth Colony governor, Myles Standish, and 39 other passengers commissioned the Mayflower Compact, the first governing document in the New World. They then explored the back shore from Truro to Eastham before moving on to Plymouth Harbor for greater shelter. Plymouth Rock is merely an invention of the Chamber of Commerce. In fact, there is no official reference to the Pilgrims landing on a rock at Plymouth; it is not mentioned in Edward Winslow's eminent *Mourt's Relation*, written in 1622, nor in Bradford's historic journal *Of Plymouth Plantation*, published 20 years later. The first recorded reference to the Pilgrims landing on a rock in Plymouth, in fact, came 121 years later.

What is an undeniable fact of history, however, is that my mother's favorite Eastham beach, First Encounter on Cape Cod Bay, is where Pilgrims first encountered Native Americans in the New World in a hostile introduction. Arrows flew, shots were fired, and all safely scattered. Historians speculate that the Native Americans might have been responding to the starving Pilgrims' discovery a month earlier in Truro of a lifesaving cache of buried corn.

"And sure it was God's good providence that we found this corn for else we know not how we should have done," Bradford wrote in his journal.

My mother loved First Encounter, a place of retreat, a refuge to gather her thoughts or watch a blazing red sun at dusk dip into the bay to be extinguished like a candle. She equally savored Coast Guard Beach in Eastham, my favorite ocean retreat—site of the old Life Saving Station whose courageous crews patrolled the stormy shoreline in the 1800s in search of shipwrecked sailors. Since the wreck of the *Sparrow-Hawk* in 1626, more than 3,000 ships have run aground in the treacherous shoals of the Great Outer Beach. The Pilgrims were a near miss here. On November 9, 1620, the *Mayflower*, 65 days out from Plymouth, England, made landfall off Coast Guard Beach, caught on the shifting shoals. Far off course from its intended destination of what is now Northern Virginia, a miraculous change in wind freed the *Mayflower* to sail north to Provincetown.

History abounds off Coast Guard Beach.

At my mother's bearing, during the spring, summer, and fall of the early '70s, often after an ocean storm, I walked south along Coast Guard Beach about two miles to a snug, windblown 21-foot-by-16-foot, two-room beach shack with a frugal wooden writing desk overlooking the surf. It was called the "Outermost House" venerated in the classic Henry Beston nature book of that name, chronicling a lone year on the Great Outer Beach. A Harvard-educated writer and naturalist, Beston built the cottage in 1925 mostly from scrap drift wood, dubbing it the "Fo'castle," given its ten windows and commanding presence atop a high dune overlooking the open Atlantic that offered the sense of being aboard a ship. In 1964, the cottage was preserved as a national literary landmark "wherein he [Beston] sought the great truth and found it in the nature of man." My mother, after reading the *Outermost House*, first took me there. I was possessed, and returned alone often to peer inside at the crude, wooden writing desk, and to sit on the outside porch and contemplate the isolated nature around me. It was here that I decided to pursue a life of writing. My mom, as she had many times before and would again, led me to a solitary place in life.

In Beston's writing, you could hear the sound of the sea. "Listen to the surf," Beston wrote. "Really lend it your ears, and you will hear in it a world of sounds: hollow boomings and heavy roarings, great watery tumblings and tramplings, long hissing seethes, sharp, rifle-shot reports, splashes, whispers, the grinding undertone of stones, and sometimes vocal sounds that might be the half-heard talk of people in the sea."

Like my mother, I felt at peace here, a calm shattered by the Great Storm of February 1978 with sustained winds of close to 100 miles an hour and an overwash of nearly 15 feet that swept the Fo'castle out to sea. The loss was devastating, but a fitting burial for a place that had brought us closer together.

Our relationship wasn't always that way. I was close to my mother growing up, but distant over time. She clearly saw a lot of my father in me, and often channeled her angst toward him through me, more as years progressed; then it turned to rage. Perhaps she felt comfortable directing it at me. In some ways, I was the embodiment of my father: male, selfish, and clueless. I was an easy mark.

By the 1990s, there had been a tidal surge in our relationship, as my mom's shifting moods were vented more and more in my direction. Looking back, I know now that she was reaching out in fear and anger over what was happening to her, and yet, I was pulling away, never grasping the moment.

"I'm your mother!" she would scream at me repeatedly, as if to convince herself. I thought at the time she was pulling rank, but she was just seeking reinforcement. I never saw it coming. We had chilling moments of conflicts, both of us pushing back at one another with the force of a wave crashing a sturdy bluff. Neither of us moved.

My 40th birthday was a ceasefire, a surprise birthday for which everyone dressed as a person of history. My mom came as Rose Kennedy, attired in a dark wig with all the graciousness of a Kennedy; it was an appropriate rendering, given their collective love and respect for family. Wrote Kennedy in her 1974 autobiography, *Times to Remember*: "I looked on child rearing not only as a work of love and a duty, but as a profession that was fully as interesting and challenging as any honorable profession in the world, and one that demanded the best I could bring to it ... " My dad, in contrast, came as Panama's Manuel Noriega, the Latin strongman accused of drug trafficking, racketeering, and money laundering. Dad had filled condoms with sugar looking like hanging bags of cocaine tied to the buttons of his shirt. It was an unforgettable night of family and friends laughing, drinking, and dancing. It was one of the last times that I remember my mother fully articulate and bountifully engaged. She wrote candidly in a birthday scrapbook of recollections, a testament that defined our relationship:

I remember when Greg in the Third Grade served his first Sunday Mass as an altar boy. He was with a more experienced altar boy, and somehow got confused and ended up on the side of the altar with the bells. In those days, bells were a big thing at Mass. Greg was terrified. At the time of the consecration of the host, no bells rang. Greg froze! The other altar boy kept telling Greg to ring the bells. Still no bells. Repeating this several times had little effect, except Greg did pick up the bells; he just couldn't ring them. He froze again. No bells. Finally, the exacerbated priest, host in hand, turned and yelled at Greg, 'Ring the God damn bells!' At that point, Greg started ringing like St. Patrick's Cathedral, and didn't stop until the priest turned around once more and said, 'Greg, stop the bells!' The nuns were all laughing, the congregation was laughing. I was crying.

We had each other's back, just didn't know it at the time. Mom reminded me that night of the time I was asked to read a scripture verse at my brother Paul's wedding. Typically, I lost my place in the reading, but instead of panicking, I relied on my altar boy training and earlier counsel from her to ad lib when your back is against the wall. So, I *ad libitum* the balance of the passage—tossing in a few "thou(s)" and some fire and brimstone. No one caught on, but my mom. When I returned to the pew, she patted me on the knee and said, "Nice work: Matthew, Mark, Luke, and John would be some proud!"

Ad lib was to become a cornerstone in our lives; in the months and years to come, it would become more apparent, as I began experiencing similar moments of confusion, recurrent memory loss, trouble at times finding the right words, problems with balance and problem solving, and a pendulum of emotions that I couldn't manage. We talked about it; the symptoms wouldn't wane for either of us. Following my mother's example, I just ignored the signs, focusing instead on work, my spouse, children, and friends—a focus, however, that fades as the disease evolves and one is wedged in isolation.

As a caregiver for my mother and breadwinner of the family, I found it difficult to ask for help. My role had been on the giving, not receiving, end, and to reverse roles was an admission of failure. I preferred, like my mother, to keep to familiar patterns of behavior, the routine, rather than concede the awful changes in play. I was trying desperately to hold onto who I was for as long as possible, knowing the disease ultimately would rob that from me.

We were both feeling terrible isolation. My mother had only two good friends on the Cape, my father notwithstanding— Tom and Mary Collins, an affable retired couple, who lived directly across the street on Cestaro Way. Mom spent much time with them. They didn't seem to mind her quirkiness. They met for lunch, for talk, for end of the day cocktails on occasion. One afternoon about ten years ago in early fall, Tom came over to the house to chat with my mom. My dad had gone for the New York papers. Tom and my mother talked about family, politics, sports, and anything else you could squeeze into a half-hour visit. When the conversation ended, he turned to my mother as he walked out the door.

"You know, Ginny, I've lived a good, full life," he observed. "As far as I'm concerned, if the Lord wants to take me, He can have me any time He wants!"

Tom gently hugged my mom. She waved to him as he walked across Cestaro in his characteristic enthusiastic gait. He opened his front door, stepped across the threshold, then dropped dead instantly. Bang. Massive heart attack. The Lord often takes us at our word.

Mom was devastated. She was never the same. She let go a bit that day. Within a few months, Mary had moved back to

Connecticut, and Mom was alone again. I noticed a softening in our relationship. Beyond my father, absorbed in his own medical issues, she now had no friends on the Cape, and thus turned to me, emotionally and for chores around the house, as she faced down her demons.

****

I always had thought of myself as Mr. Green Jeans, the genial sidekick to Captain Kangaroo. Mr. Green Jeans always performed ably with hand puppets, talked to Grandfather Clock, introduced live animals, taught little children to care for the Earth, but he couldn't fix squat. Neither could I. Accepting of this, my mom kept it simple, just asking me in late spring to install the bulky window air conditioner in the living room, replace screens with storm windows in the fall, paint the outside trim, clean the gutters, and wrap the hoses for storage. I think she just wanted me around the house to talk. She was lonely, and when she wasn't talking, she just stared out of the window. Blank stares, as if she were on Pluto.

On a late Sunday afternoon in October 2000, I finally started to get it. Mom asked me to take her to the bank; I wasn't sure why. She said she needed to use the ATM. A banker earlier in life and one who had used a cash card often, she told me she was having difficulty with the machine. She couldn't figure out how to use it; tried several times. She was completely out of sorts.

"Greg, I'm scared," she told me in the bank parking lot. "I can't do this anymore. I get confused all the time. I need someone to talk to. Will you help me? Please don't tell your father!"

I will never forget that day. The sky was gray, the wind was blowing on shore, and there was a penetrating chill in the air.

"Sure, Mom," I said, beginning to realize her inner fear of losing control. "We're good now. We're just good, Mom."

I never looked back on the relationship, my anger over her rants at me; I only looked forward now. I was Mr. Green Jeans, wholly useless, yet destined to be a caregiver. Hand me the Phillips screwdriver! Just tell me which end is up.

****

Confusion in time gave way to chaos. My mother began putting garbage in the trunk of the car—forgetting to take it to the dump, opting to horde. The maggots and stench were revolting, yet my siblings and I were reticent to deal head-on with it. Mom began hiding money in the house from my father, wads of it; she slept in her clothes; made up words for lack of recall; often refused to shower; and grabbed for liquid soap at times to brush her teeth. Then there were the "menu issues." My dad in his wheelchair would ask for ice cream for dessert, and she'd serve him eggs, sunny-side up. The behavior upset me and equally distressed my father, who observed it nightly. At first, we collectively passed it off as a change-of-life transition, but the shift intensified.

After all the anguish in our relationship, my mother and I were on parallel tracks. She was years ahead of me, but I could see her in the distance, not sure where she was headed. Yet, I followed. Then one day, my ticket to Pluto arrived by way of a blissful bicycle ride from Brewster. On a postcard-perfect day, I had taken my son, Conor, and his friend, Ryan White, both about 12 at the time, on a trek along the Cape Cod Rail Trail to Eastham, about a 15-mile ride, to visit my mother—a pastoral passage beside sparkling cranberry bogs, lush meadows, saltwater marshes, and fresh water ponds. In all ways, it was a cleansing, majestic Cape Cod day. Mom, however, was more muddled than usual. With the temperature inching toward 80, she scolded all of us for not wearing winter coats. To take the "chill" off, she insisted the boys don these heavy, oversized sweatshirts from a spare bedroom closet, largesse from winters past. They balked at first, but sensing her resolve, I instructed them to oblige.

"Mom's right," I summoned. "It's cold out."

Conor, having witnessed corresponding episodes in the past, concurred, and Ryan graciously consented. The second we peddled out of the driveway, turning left on Cestaro Way toward the bike trail, the boys ripped off the sweatshirts and tossed them at me.

"No way, we're not wearing these things!" Conor declared.

I thanked the boys for being good sports, and draped the heavy sweatshirts across the handlebars of my bike as we headed back to Brewster, taking in a panorama of primal nature. I was euphoric, in the Zen, incredibly at peace. I felt like a kid again, and plied the trail in full speed far ahead of Conor and Ryan. Faster, faster! The wind was soothing. In the moment, I recalled that, as a youth, I had prided myself on riding a red, three-speed Schwinn racer, no handed! And like a child, I wasn't wearing a helmet that day. For 30 seconds, I peddled back in time, a kaleidoscope of images from youth: Rye Beach, the ball field at Disbrow Park, town marina, and out to the American Yacht Club where you could see the Manhattan skyline and Twin Towers in the distance. Then, as abrupt as a clap of thunder, the imagery shifted. I sensed something awry. In horrifying slow motion, what seemed like frame-by-frame, I witnessed the sweatshirts on the handlebars slip slowly into the spokes. My bike, at full gallop, stopped on a dime, and I was hurled head first over the handlebars about 15 feet into the air, but with the presence of mind at least to shield my left hand over my forehead before impact. I hit the tarmac with the force, it seemed, of a .45 caliber bullet, the impact cutting deep into my knuckles right through to the bone. On the second bounce, my face hit the pavement in a pool of blood. I was numb, out of body, yet felt something cold pouring down my face. As I finally stood up, I must have looked like the lead role in a Bela Lugosi movie; in pure fright, Conor and Ryan sprinted off into the woods. Two Samaritans sitting on a nearby back deck came to my aid, and collected the kids. The rest is fleeting; a half hour later I was rushed to Cape Cod

Hospital in an ambulance, sirens ablaze. After multiple stitches to the head and left hand, I was discharged.

Little did I know that I had unleashed a monster.

12

Passing the Baton

THE LEGENDARY TRACK STAR JESSE OWENS FACED A MONSTER. In the summer of 1936, just years before the start of World War II, demon Adolf Hitler and his Nazi faithful were goose-stepping across Eastern Europe. At the Berlin Olympics, Hitler sought to showcase purported Aryan superiority and chastised the U.S. for engaging gifted African Americans, whom he termed "sub-humans," to compete against his Aryan Nation. Owens stared the demons down, winning four gold medals: 100 meters, 200 meters, long jump, and 4x100 meter relay, the final affront to Hitler, making Owens the most decorated athlete of the 1936 Olympics. Owens ran the first leg of the relay in a record 39.8 seconds, picking up a two-meter lead, and resolutely passing the baton to Ralph Metcalfe, an African American who was the fastest human from 1932 to 1934, and later served in the U.S. Congress. A purposeful passing, at this critical moment in time, propelled Metcalfe to a four-meter lead, the measure of success. Foy Draper, who ran the third leg, maintained the lead, and 100-yard world record holder Frank Wykoff, with baton firmly in stride lengthened the winning margin to 15 meters, beating his Italian counterpart, Tullio Gonnelli.

An efficacious passing of the baton in a relay race is as elemental as lacing up a pair of running shoes, and has relevance in the race against Alzheimer's. Timing is critical. When a runner hits a mark on the track, usually a small triangle, the awaiting runner—on cue and face forward—opens a backward hand, and after a few strides, the lead runner has caught up and exchanges the baton. Often, the lead runner will shout "*stick!*" several times as a signal for the awaiting runner, glancing behind, to put out a hand. Passing the baton has significance on many fronts—on a track, at home, at work, in disease, and into eternity. In the relay race of life, one can't run alone. You sprint your leg as best as possible, then hand off with precision, letting others carry you as they can. Looking back, I realize now that my mother, in trying to outrun Alzheimer's, was yelling at me, "*Stick … stick … stick!*"

****

You can see eternity from Eastham and elsewhere. Ever look between two facing mirrors, at home, in a barbershop or a beauty salon? You face a seemingly endless line of images fading into the distance. In principle, it's called "looking into infinity." Each mirror reflects the image into the other mirror, bouncing these reflections back and forth into infinity—gateways, some speculate, to parallel universes. If you squint, you might see Pluto and beyond.

My mom was a mirror, preparing me as only a mother could to see through her lens into infinity and pass the baton. The day after I was released from Cape Cod Hospital after the bike accident, she arrived early in the morning at my house in Brewster with bandages and rubbing alcohol in hand. In her altered state, she was rushing over to stop the bleeding. I was covered in hospital bandages with more than 20 stitches to the face and hands, all washed up, and yet, she insisted on cleaning the wounds. Her signals were confused. She was still my mother, knew it, and proceeded to clean the bandages with rubbing alcohol. I let her, realizing she was living in the moment, and at that moment, so was I. She was my mother, even in her Alzheimer's, and I desperately wanted to be her son.

I hope my children, as this disease progresses, will allow me to be their father. It is vital for those with Alzheimer's to connect with the past, the long-term memories and relationships. The short term is a flash.

Parallel universes between my mother and me collided after my accident. We were over the handlebars, and together could see into infinity.

****

But one must squint to see into infinity, stretching the mind. The word, with mathematical definition, has derivation in the Latin word *infinitas,* meaning "unbounded," a noun with roots in the ancient Greek word *apeiros*, which translates to endless. In my mother's final years, I had endless conversations with her, including regular Sunday night *tête-à-têtes* at the dinner table with my folks in Eastham beside a large picture window overlooking a patch of scrub oak and pine, bent from winter winds into forms that stretch the imagination. The curved oak table with sturdy legs and high-back Queen Anne chairs forced one to sit upright. Bought at a discount home improvement center, it still had the emotive feel of a medieval round table, not because it resembled an antique, but because a Prodigal Son now had occasion for final wisdom from his parents. I cherish those moments, some of them painful, all of them imbedded in my soul.

Dad, as usual, drove the conversation with pounding, penetrating queries, challenging me on politics, sports, religion, sibling rivalries, and just about any other subject one is not supposed to talk about in public. Mom was quick, as she could, on rebuttal. It kept her mind challenged and active. She deflected my dad's barbs like a veteran hockey goalie, which were meant more to make her think than overreact.

My cerebral training early on was served up in Rye at the family dinner table, a relic today. All ten of us were seated on Brookdale Place on Sundays around a thick plank of mahogany. We were akin to knights in shining armor; only our swords were stainless steel, barely sharp enough to cut the overcooked beef, and our breastplates were paper napkins slung from the collar. Still, we were a force. My folks would query us, like a pop quiz, about our lives, our friends, attitudes, beliefs, and trouble on the horizon, just to get inside our pointy little heads. I thought of the exercise, at the time, as a holy inquest, but as I grew older, I enjoyed the banter. It brought us all together. But there were exceptions. Like the time when my older sister Maureen called me out in high school, lobbed a grenade under the table, for my dating on the sly a well-endowed, exceptionally attractive coed several years older than I was.

"So, Greg, why don't you tell us about it?" said Maureen, the self-appointed "Mother Superior" of the family.

Dad dropped his fork. Mom glowered at me. And I stared intently at Maureen in an attempt to burn her retinas, but they were blocks of ice.

"So, what's this all about?" Dad asked.

The sizzling meatloaf before me that I had so coveted had all the appeal now of a pair of worn sneakers after a sweaty basketball drill.

"Oh," I said lamely, "We just went to the movies together. I think it was the *Ten Commandments*."

"Yeah," Maureen interjected between mouthfuls of mashed potatoes, "Thou shalt not sin!"

"That's enough," Dad declared, shutting down the discourse. I wasn't sure if he was disgusted or proud of me.

Mom nodded in a way that said firmly: *Greg, you can do better.* The look alone served to bring me up short, but those words have become a mantra throughout my life. I still envision my mother urging me on. In the moment, the exchange that day was discomforting, yet enlightening. Looking back, such wordplay reinforces the family dinner table as a forum for in-your-face instruction, edification, and for unforgettable family bonding.

Such illumination continued decades later at the more intimate dinner table on the Cape. Observing my mom's frontal assault on Alzheimer's, the wisdom was abundantly enriching. Perspective has a way of cutting through a disease. Every Sunday at twilight after leaving Willy's Gym in Orleans, I drove alone to Eastham for introspection with my parents. The drive was a timeline of sorts, passing Town Cove to the starboard where schooners once delivered their consignment from the Old World; Salt Pond, a brackish estuary, rich with shellfish, that empties into the Atlantic; Evergreen Cemetery where the markers date back to the time of the Pilgrims, and where my parents eventually would rest; and across from the cemetery, Arnold's Lobster and Clam Bar, a family favorite where the sweet, salty aroma of fresh seafood off the dock wafts across the tombstones. Arnold's, formerly Betty's Beach Box, is run by a childhood friend and Pilgrim descendent, Nate Nickerson, a.k.a. Nathan Atwood Nickerson III, whose *Mayflower* forbearers settled the Cape. Arnold's was my mother's favorite eating hole; she always enjoyed talking with Nicky. Since birth, he has known the difference between a steamer and a quahog, and probably could pronounce the word *in utero.*

Such distinction was lost in time on my mother. A quahog, to her, could have been a kitchen utensil—a knife or something sharp to stick into an electrical socket, as she often tried. We had to hide the knives. One day, she noticed the kitchen paper towel rack was empty; staring at the exposed cardboard tube, she knew it should be covered with something white, so she laid pieces of bread over the tube as if hanging out clothes to dry. The slide continued with both parents. The dinner table reinforced their decline. At times, my mother served my dad coffee grinds on toast. He never let on in front of me, nor did he want to embrace the stony reality. That bothered me and my siblings terribly. In retrospect, I believe he was trying to protect my mother from reality, as he began his own fearful, slow slide into dementia himself, complicated by the throes of circulation disease and prostate cancer. It was a shit show.

At first, none of us saw the warning signs of Alzheimer's. We were all numb to it: my mother's memory loss, challenges in planning and with problem solving, difficulty completing familiar tasks, confusion with time and place, trouble understanding visual images, problems finding the right words, inability to retrace steps, poor judgment, withdrawal, swings in mood and personality, and finally, intense rage.

In the fall of 2007, reality was sinking in. At the dinner table, my parents and I talked more intensely about family, politics, and life; we talked about religion, eschatology, about God, a genderless definition of all-love, and about facing the Almighty one day. I told them several times that something wasn't right in my head. Dad dismissed it, but Mom always tried to instill courage in me.

"You must have courage," she counseled. "Never give in!"

In the final months, our dinner table discussions centered around topics we had never entertained before. End-of-life stuff. My father, now in a wheelchair with little use of his legs, waxed on about the genius of Roosevelt Democrats, the need to care for the disadvantaged, the moral obligation to pursue a passion in life that made the world just a bit better, and he probed knotty questions about what happens to you when you die. A rock-ribbed Catholic, who had lost both his parents in childhood, he feared death, and like many of us, wasn't quite sure of what awaited him on the other side. He was deathly afraid.

Mom seemed to embrace it.

Many years ago, I had a dream about death, one of what was to be several. In the dream, my father had passed away. He was in Heaven. No longer confined to a wheelchair, he was sprinting like a high school tailback, with jet-black hair combed straight back. I told my parents about it over the dinner table on September 16, 2007. I remember the day.

"Was I running to Mom?" Dad asked.

"No," I said. "You were running to your parents."

He paused.

"Was Mom there?" he asked.

"No," I said, knowing the implications of the response. "She hadn't left yet."

"Not my time!" Mom evoked with confidence.

And it wasn't. My father was to die first on January 5, 2008, my brother Tim's birthday. Mom died four months later on May 21; she was buried on my sister Lauren's birthday. So much for birthdays.

In that moment, collectively, we were well into the stages of grief: shock; denial and isolation; anger; bargaining; depression; testing; acceptance; and hope. We hadn't turned the corner yet on hope.

The dictionary defines hope as desire with anticipation; scripture describes it as faith in a seed form. All of us were in need of watering. Mom knew her time, but always held her tongue. Liberal in some ways, conservative in others, walking lockstep with traditional spiritual values, she often said she regretted not speaking her mind on more occasions. It was a sad commentary, given her diminishing state of intellect. Sadly, women a generation ago were to be seen, but not heard. They carried babies, cared for children, and were the fabric that held families together like glue. Imagine what we all could have learned had we listened more.

I listened too late, learning far more from my mother's assail on death than from her wisdom and duty to family. I whiffed at that. In contrast to the culture today of self-indulgence, the mothers in the Greatest Generation were selfless in devotion, not out of diffidence, but in maternal instinct—a promise of love, beyond the capacity of most men. Even in Alzheimer's, the love persisted.

My mother in her bruising 15- to 20-year progression of Alzheimer's, refused to lie down. She carried us at times, like a soldier in Patton's army, when she wasn't quite sure what planet she was on. I watched in awe, as did my sisters and brothers. Mom's role had changed, and would change again. Yet, none of us wanted to concede the obvious: our mother was slowly sliding off the face of the Earth, pulled into the metaphorical orbits of Pluto and Sedna.

The nursing of my father took its toll on Mom's health. Her memory continued to fade, like cedar shingles bleached by the sun; her rage intensified; she didn't recognize family members and friends at times; she wandered and drifted; she was scared. But she cared, as best she could, for my father and for the rest of us. The ancient Greeks called it *Agape*, the purest form of unconditional love, far purer than *Eros* (physical passion), *Philia* (brotherly love), and *Storge* (affection). Mom wanted to hold to her role as wife and mother, but roles were changing. She was fighting demons, forever pushing back against monsters in the shadows.

In 2007, my dad was back in Cape Cod Hospital for a second, life-threatening circulation bypass surgery, and she stood with him again against all odds. It was her final stand. She was about done. Over lunch at a restaurant on Hyannis Harbor, walking distance from the hospital, she took my wife, Mary Catherine, aside in an emotional breakdown, and within my earshot, she growled with venom, *"I hate him. I hate him. I hate him. I just haaaaate him!"*

She wasn't referring to my father, but venting rage against me, perceived in the moment as the surrogate husband. She was reluctant to confront my father in his suffering, dutiful to the end. The elephant was under the tent. It consumed the space, and it just blew me away.

The tent flaps opened wide and led to Epoch nursing home in Brewster where my father was sent for rehabilitation, and Mom followed because she could no longer safely be alone and because she wanted to be with Dad. They were side-by-side in separate beds in an antiseptic, sterile first-floor room. It was difficult to tell which one was the patient. Mom was somnolent, and when she spoke, made little sense—a chilling contrast of a little child, then a raging adult. The brain wasn't firing. Signals were crossed. The scene was an awakening, a cold shower, for the siblings who had visited; they were appalled at Mom's plummet. Dad was ever distrustful, fearing in his advancing paranoia that we were attempting to commit him to the nursing home. The irony was that Mom needed to be cared for far more than he; she was out of sorts to the point of insentience, yet laser sharp with long-term memory about the particulars of her life and family. The following day when the devoted Epoch staff took her by the hand to the library filled with four walls of books, they asked her what she wanted to read. The nurses told me later that she scanned the shelves for 15 minutes, and then pulled out two books.

"I think I'll read these," she finally said, not grasping the title or author.

The books she chose were *Secrets in the Sand* and *A Guide to Nature on Cape Cod and the Islands*—two books of mine published many years ago, and two books that she had kept in her living room in Eastham.

"They just felt comfortable in her hands," the nurse told me later.

At Epoch, it was clear to presiding physician Dr. Robert Harmon that my mother was on tilt, moving from mid-stage Alzheimer's to end-stage, still she wanted to be the wife and mother. Dr. Harmon called for family intervention, a conference at Epoch that looped in siblings over the phone who could not attend. It was a disaster of a family conference, as it might be with other large families. Many of the siblings, in this College of Cardinals, were at different end points—from positions of denial, to circumspection, to anger, as Dr. Robert Harmon sought to bring us to a place of irrefutable reality: Alzheimer's was consuming Virginia Brown O'Brien, and there was nothing that any of us could do about it. Nothing.

In the weeks to come, I sought, as my parents' designated Power of Attorney and Healthcare Proxy—a position of impotence in a large family—to find common ground among the siblings, something similar to striking peace on the Gaza Strip. The warring factions, with all good intentions, were split. The girls justifiably wanted Mom protected in a nursing home, and the boys sought to keep my parents together at home. We were split in a moment of crisis, and the crevasse was widening. Deep into confusion myself and privately questioning my logic, I cast the defining vote. Mom and Dad would stay at home, here on Cestaro Way, the dead-end street.

My parents returned to Eastham the following week with the commander-in-chief, holding tight to the concept of hunkering down in the cottage below the tracer bullets. My dad's survival instinct, motivated by fear, was to ride out the storm with my mother. And so, at his unrelenting direction, we hired 24/7 in-home healthcare to be paid out of his Pan Am pension fund at a nosebleed rate of $25,000-a-month for both parents. These were well-meaning, dedicated professional caregivers, but do the math.

It was a free fall, medically and financially, two Black Hawks down! Clear the decks. "Only the dead have seen the end of war," Plato once said; a declaration that opened Ridley Scott's classic 1991 movie. We all sat back in horror, as if observing in slow motion a horrific air-show crash—my father in a wheelchair, with internal bleeding and no use of his legs; Mom, in short circuit, with little use of her intellect. Regularly, I called them at night, just to check in, and when no one answered, I would race in a fire drill to Eastham, sometimes at 11 pm, thinking I would find them dead, only to realize my mom forgot to hang up the phone.

The reality was debilitating for my brothers and sisters who lived off-Cape, as it would be for any family with such a commute. Over time, Mom's rage and Dad's incessant crusade for survival accelerated, for various and incongruous reasons. I tried to underscore the point one night over the Sunday dinner table, but Dad wasn't getting the fact that his wife of 60 years was slowly drifting out, that I was drifting as well, and both of us were getting angry.

Regrettably, my father, once my hero, never read Ernest Hemingway's *The Sun Also Rises*: "You can't get away from yourself by moving from one place to another." The trip from Epoch back to Eastham changed nothing. The thoughts of collateral damage stunned me, as I confronted my own demons. I started shifting fidelities. I had no choice. Mom was alone and vulnerable.

****

October is a special time on Cape Cod and the Islands. The sun rises later in the morning and sets lower on the horizon, yet high enough to light up the emerald salt-marsh grass. Indian summer is in play, a period of unseasonably warm, dry weather, a bonus for the locals. The Cape in fall is heated by the warmth of water surrounding this narrow spit of sand; consequently, summer is longer here, and spring generally arrives for a day in early June.

As the sun set over Cape Cod Bay on Sunday, October 14,

2007, Columbus Day weekend, I headed to Eastham after restarting my brain at the gym. I was in full flush on the way to Eastham, reflecting on my parents, their fading health, and my conflicting instinct about keeping them together at the cottage, for better or for worse.

****

My father—months from dying and he knew it—was particularly prickly that night with incessant pain, internal bleeding, and a continued breakdown of the body and mind. Dad clearly was on tilt; my mom couldn't think at all; and the professional caregiver at the house, God bless him, had trouble with the English language. Mom, that night, had served pickles sprinkled on Cheerios for dinner; last time I had that was in college after smoking some recreational dope. All the ingredients were in place for a blow-up of denial when I arrived. My father, fully paranoid, had assumed I had come to take him and my mother to a nursing home. He was itching for a fight. We were at the anger and bargaining stage of grief.

"*Tell your brothers and sisters that we're doing fine here, and that we don't need your damn help!*" he bellowed. "*You can leave now, son! We don't need you!*"

"Dad, I'm just here to see Mom," I said quietly.

"*Well, your mother doesn't want to see you either.*"

Immediately, my mother moved to a seat next to me, putting her right arm over my shoulders. She never said a word. Perhaps a sign she was switching allegiances.

My dad persisted. "*The bodies are still warm here, Greg. Go home. You haven't done a damn thing for us. So, just go away, go A-W-A-Y!*"

"Dad," I said. "I get it; you're scared of dying; I get that, but Mom is very sick, and she needs our help."

"*You've done nothing for us, Greg. Ever! Nothing!*"

The words cut to my heart. They were delivered in my

father's fear, but I was done with it.

"*Dad,*" I screamed in a spray of expletives. "*Do you think you're the first person in the world to die? Dying sucks, Dad. I imagine, it freakin' sucks, but we all die some day.*"

I paused for a second, which seemed like minutes, fully aware of what I was about to shout: "*SO WHY DON'T YOU TRY NOW TO DIE WITH SOME DIGNITY, DAD, AND TAKE CARE OF MOM ALONG THE WAY!*"

There was deafening silence; you could count heartbeats. We were all crying, and the elephant in the room had consumed the oxygen. We were emotionally gasping. Gabriel, my parent's faithful caregiver, intervened as a messenger angel. He stepped in and separated me from my father, directing me to a back room. Still traumatized by what I had just said, I followed Gabriel, and Mom followed me. The torch had been passed. Gabriel brought me a glass of water, an act of kindness still imbedded in my memory. He made no judgments, and then returned to my father, as any caregiver should.

Mom and I then sat quietly in the back room, surrounded by the memories of family photographs—her mother growing up on a horse farm in Brooklyn, my dad as a handsome Navy lieutenant, her children as young kids on Nauset Beach. She was still crying.

"I'm scared," she said. "What's happening to me?"

"Mom," I said, looking into her eyes. "I know the pain. I feel some of it. You're not alone. We are all here for you."

I pointed with my right index finger to her forehead. "Do you remember that little girl who grew up on the West Side of Manhattan, do you remember the little girl who went to the French convent school, then grew up, got married, and had ten children?"

"Yes," she said, intently staring at me.

"Well that little girl, Mom, that wonderful mother, hasn't left yet; she's still inside you. Believe that!"

"*REALLY?*" she asked drawing out the word, sobbing now, perhaps the first time she admitted she was lost in space and not coming back.

"Yes," I affirmed. "And that little girl will never leave you as long as you fight until you can't fight anymore. You understand that, Mom? Do you understand that?"

"I do," she said definitively.

That's all I needed to hear.

We walked back hand-in-hand into the living room. Dad had calmed down, and Gabriel was hovering next to him.

"I love you, Dad," I said as I walked out the door. "But you really pissed me off tonight. You're better than that! Much better than that."

The following day at 7 am, Dad called me.

"I'm sorry," he said. The contrition was short, to the point, deeply sincere, and duly noted.

It was behind us now. Finally, we were all on the same page.

The roles clearly had changed, but it was a downhill slope, reminding me of the Outer Limits run at Killington, Vt. I was hitting red marker poles along the way, collectively in the depression, reflection, and the loneliness of grief, a changing of the guard for a fate that lay ahead. I never confided in Mary Catherine about this; wasn't sure she could or would go there. Still not sure. And who would blame her? I was looking inward, trying to protect what I could, a matter of duty as a husband and father for as long as I could.

13

Angels Unawares

M Y MOTHER LOVED YELLOW, THE COLOR OF THE MIND and the intellect, the third chakra of the solar plexus, representing personal power and spark. Yellow is the hue, most visible of all, of memory, hope, happiness, and enlightenment. Yellow inspires the dreamer; encourages the seeker. My mom's rapture with yellow was an upward, heavenly turn in the stages of grief.

Yellow is a color of angels, and in scripture it symbolizes a change for the better. Mom believed in angels. So do I. The word, derived from the ancient Latin *"Angelus"* translated "messenger" or "envoys," resonates with peace. And in the throes of Alzheimer's, that's pure gold; if you scratch below the surface of life, messengers may abound, as Hebrews 13:2 counsels: "Be not forgetful to entertain strangers for thereby some have entertained angels unawares."

My mother, I believe, entertained angels unawares. Seven months before her death, in late fall 2007, she became obsessed with the color yellow. She saw yellow everywhere, mostly yellow cars. All she talked about was yellow. I dismissed the thought outright. Weeks later, driving my mother to Brown's Superette, across from the Eastham Windmill, the oldest working gristmill on the Cape, she exclaimed, "Greg, do you see that yellow car? Look, there's another one, *and another one!*"

Holy snikes, I was seeing yellow now, myself. In time, so was my brother Tim, who lives in Guilford, Conn., and faithfully visited my parents frequently. So, Tim opted to buy a yellow Jeep Wrangler. My mother was thrilled every time he drove into the driveway, somewhat of a second coming. Taking a cue from my younger brother, I also bought a yellow Jeep. We were heaven on wheels—Mom's angels-at-arms. She loved driving in our Jeeps, like a kid on an amusement ride at Playland in Rye. My brother still has his yellow Jeep. So do I. And I'm taking mine to the grave.

As a New England November gave way to December, the days were tersely shorter—a sundowner effect for all. The sun, lower in the sky at the vernal equinox, now dipped into Cape Cod Bay at 4:09 pm, as the hourglass sand of my parents' lives were slipping through our fingers. Alzheimer's was bearing down on my mother in the final stage of the disease; Dad was succumbing to his circulation disorders, the progressing effects of prostate cancer, and advancing dementia; and I was adrift on days, off my mooring, tethered to a lifeline, a loving family. We were all living on the edge of faith, with a bit of attitude from Alfred E. Neuman, the red-headed urchin of iconic *Mad Magazine;* the kid with the blissful grin: *"What, me worry?"*

My mother was worried, but endured the disease resolutely as it moved to full bout. The progression was much like watching paint dry on a moist day, ever steady and slow, but the results were unassailable. Still, she functioned as a dutiful military nurse, endeavoring to care for her husband, as other wives of this generation had selflessly done with spouses. Somehow, these women were lost in the headlines. They prevailed against all odds. But where were the medals and headlines for them?

There were yet more crisis runs to Cape Cod Hospital in December. Responding to my father's critical internal bleeding and the unrelenting strain of holding a thought wore my mother to a nub. I followed in tow. We were at the tipping point—an irreversible moment in time, like a glass of fine Bordeaux Cabernet Sauvignon spilling over onto a white-linen table cloth. Standing up the glass will not retrieve the wine, nor will it remove the crimson stain. My mom was packing for Pluto, and Dad, forever the Navy man, was setting up deck chairs on his *Titanic*, awaiting a rescue that would never come. The siblings were apoplectic.

My father, meanwhile, kept his humor. After one of his many Lazarus-like resurrections, he barked when the phone rang at home, *"If that's Nickerson Funeral Home, tell them I'm not ready yet!"*

Mom was ready, but didn't know it. Rudderless and adrift, she fought alongside my father—perhaps fearing being left behind, maybe out of instinct. Dad was her rock; we were her kids. She wanted it that way, never ignoring the chain of command. While Alzheimer's can ravage a mind, it cannot erase instinct, the capacity to acquire knowledge without interference or reason. Instinct has history in the Latin verb, *intueri*, "to look inside." My mother taught me to look inside, to turn over the rocks, particularly when one cannot fathom the reality, the certainty, of what is happening on the surface.

Certainty was served up bedside to my parents at Cape Cod Hospital on November 11, 2007, a month before my father's 85th birthday and about eight weeks before his death. Dr. Alice Daley, a skilled internist and compassionate woman who had closely studied my parents' medical records, discerned it was time for a come-to-Jesus talk. Damn the denial, Dr. Daley knew life was short for both. With my dad in the prone position, my mom seated by his side and insisting she stay, anticipating the worst, and with me, a stunned observer, at the foot of the bed feeling like a voyeur, Dr. Daley gently asked my father if he was prolonging life or death: "If life is a desire to live in some quality, real or imagined, then one is prolonging life," she said. "But if life is fear of death, then one is prolonging death."

Dad, deep in the throes of his own dementia, was prolonging his death. So was my mom.

Dr. Daley, in one of the most remarkable, powerful exchanges I've ever witnessed, then asked my parents to give each other permission to die—the "working through" stage of grief.

"Virginia," she began softly, "how do you feel about Frank dying?"

In instinct, Mom rose to the occasion.

"I will miss him terribly," she said. "And that frightens me."

Sensing the moment, fully aware of my mom's state of mind, yet knowing my mother might later regret a moment lost, Dr. Daley asked her point blank, "Do you give your husband permission to die?"

The words pounded through my brain.

There was a pause, as affected as I've ever witnessed.

"Yes, I do," my mother said, tears welling up. She knew where life and death was heading for the both of them.

"Did you hear that, Frank?" Dr. Daley asked.

"I do," he replied.

"How do you feel about dying first?"

"I want to die first," my father said quietly. "I don't want to be alone. I don't want to live without Virginia. I can't handle it."

Mom reached for his hand.

Denial in the moment had given way to soul-searching truth.

Another baton had been passed in the resurrection of their relationship.

****

"Do Not Resuscitate," the forbidding acronym, DNR, is the kiss of death. We were all raised to cherish life, and this core belief was now being called into question. A DNR was in play for both parents, a "no code," as nurses call it, a signed affidavit to respect the wishes of a natural death. And I, the Prodigal Son, "Lunchie," the guy growing up who often was missing in action, was to make the final call. Not good. It wasn't the position I had anticipated earlier in life; as a young man, I had squandered my parents' moderate means on travel, good wine, and trying in vain to sway women far above my station in life. The DNR weighed heavily on me.

The fire drills continued. After Christmas, my sister Lauren, who lives north of Boston, came for a visit one afternoon and found my parents home alone. A substitute caregiver had run to the store to pick up the *The New York Times* and *Daily News* for my dad. When my sister arrived at the cottage, my father was sitting in his wheelchair facing the wall. A horrific chain smoker, he was puffing a cigarette queued up to his oxygen tank, behavior as rash as lighting a match in a nitroglycerin factory. My mother was wandering the house, insisting no one was home. KaBOOM! We were, as a family, at ground zero, a place many Boomers have been with parents, as their own children one day will be with them.

New Year's 2008, I had hoped, would bring new promise, but faith was not of this world. My dad had made it clear to me that more ambulance runs to Cape Cod Hospital were *verboten*. He was done, and I instructed the caregivers as such. But on January 4, with Archangel Gabriel off duty, a replacement caregiver in a medical crunch freaked, and rushed my father to the hospital in an ambulance. A half hour later, Dr. Daley summoned me from a meeting in Boston. I flew down Route 3 to the Sagamore Bridge, like a seagull chasing an offshore dragger so laden with fish that the scuppers were taking on water.

Walking down the corridor of the intensive care unit, I immediately instructed the medical staff that my father was going home the next day. *Got it, tomorrow!* There would be no question about it. I then went to his room. In full horror as I walked through the door, he was even more a skeleton of himself, withered in days.

"Greg," he demanded, "What the hell's going on? I don't want to be here. I told you that! I want to be home with Mom."

"I know, Dad," I apologized. "You're going home tomorrow. I have spoken with the doctors, and you're going home."

"Good!" he said.

"And you're never coming back, Dad."

"Good..."

"And you're *never* coming back again."

"Good."

"Dad, you're *NEVER* coming back here ever again!"

In one of my father's last rational moments, he pulled his scrawny frame upright to a sitting position and addressed me as only a father could lecture a son who wasn't getting it. His body language told me to stand the freak down.

"I get it," he said as if addressing a third grader. *"I ... GET ... IT!"*

The exclamation point was a hand gesture, cupping his fingers at the middle of his breastplate, then ever so slowly, for emphasis, drawing his hand to the extremes of his shoulders.

I got it, too. They were the last words my father ever spoke to me.

The hospital dispatched my father to hospice care at home the following day. My mom, I believe, knew in her heart that we were on final watch; still not sure of time and place, frozen in the moment, but knowing the moment was at hand.

The doctors had prescribed morphine for my dad's intense pain to allow him to let go, and die with some dignity, free of his fears. I was asked to pick up his final orders at the pharmacy, and bring the morphine up to the nurses in Eastham that night. The reality was chilling. I was bringing home my father's death sentence.

****

The drive to Eastham was disorienting, unlike the Sunday rides from Willy's Gym. Random images of my folks, childhood, my brothers and sisters, flashed through my head as I pondered the past, the present, and future. Only the past held hope for us that evening, and that was now on the brink.

Entering the house through the back door, fumbling with the screen that I had never fixed properly, the cottage felt as though it had the life sucked out of it. The quiet of imminent death filled my parents' bedroom. My dad was lying motionlessly in bed, eyes open, unable to talk, still resisting. My mother, steadfast as ever in Alzheimer's, was sitting by his side, not quite sure what was about to happen, but dreading horrific change in the air.

I gave the morphine to the nurse, the mother of my daughter Colleen's close high school friend. I felt as though I was wearing the mask of an executioner.

"You need to say goodbye to your father," the nurse counseled.

"What do you mean?"

"It's time, Greg."

"Time? Time for what?" I said anxiously, "I have to call my brothers and sisters; I need to get them here."

My head was throbbing.

"There is no time left. You need to say goodbye. Your dad is ready to go home."

She stared intently at me, like the Sisters of Charity at Resurrection.

Instincts locked in. I grabbed my father's hand. My mother, without prompting from me, put her hand gently on top of mine. It just seemed, for her, the right thing to do.

There is no training, no manual, for this.

"Dad," I said looking closely into his dim brown eyes. "Shake your head if you can hear me."

He nodded his head.

"I want you to know, Dad, that we will take care of Mom, all of us. I promise!"

He shook his head.

"Dad, you are very sick, and it's time to go home."

He shook his head.

"Can you see a light, Dad, a peaceful light?"

He shook his head.

"Dad, move to the light. Embrace it. We will take care of Mom. I promise you!"

He shook his head.

"Dad," I then said, "I love you, and it's been an honor to serve you."

He shook his head.

Tears were slipping down his narrow, ashen face. Together, we were at the door of acceptance and hope, looking to infinity—my dad, my mom, and me— through facing mirrors of reality. I felt as though I was gazing through a kaleidoscope, a tunnel of reflected light and colors in patterns that both comfort and confuse. It brought me back to the innocence of childhood when all seemed right. But it wasn't tonight.

Moments later my father closed his eyes. He never opened them again.

****

The following morning, Dad was pronounced dead. He passed in peace at home just where he wanted to be, lying in his bed and shielded by the unremitting love of my mother, who lay next to him, with her arms instinctively across his chest, unsure of her reality, frightened to be left alone, but dutiful to the end.

I got the call from caregivers at 6 am and raced to the cottage. When I arrived, my mom was sitting alone at the dining room table, staring blankly out into the scrub oak forest behind the house. A cold, piercing drizzle pelted the picture window; it might as well have been a rabbit hole into the fantasy world of the Queen of Hearts and the Mad Hatter, images she had faced before and would again, months later, in the nursing home. Mom was terrified. I took her by the hand to the bedroom for final valediction. Dad was still—resting in his peace. Always the wife and mother, she sat next to him and brushed his hair back, as if preparing him for an appointment.

"Mom, Dad's dead," I said.

"I know," she replied. "I'm alone. I don't know how much longer I want to be here."

Minutes later, the crew from Nickerson Funeral Home arrived. In a small Cape Cod town, everyone knows one another, and today was no exception. The crew expressed regrets, and then carefully wrapped my father's body in a white bed linen, placing him in a long black plastic bag with a zipper. As the attendant slowly zipped the bag shut, I was overcome with the certainty of death. So was my mom. In the moment, yet knowing better, I zipped down the bag so my father could breathe. I thought my mother would want that. All in the room seemed to understand. I then instructed the funeral home crew that I would walk my father out to the hearse in the stretcher. It seemed like the right thing to do.

"Mom, don't worry," I said. "Dad's not leaving here alone!"

Putting the stretcher, feet first, into the back of the hearse, I reached down and kissed my father on the forehead. I zipped up the bag. Dad was safely home now.

****

Mom was left behind and lost in the crushing wake of his death. My father was waked days later at the Nickerson Funeral Home in the center of the snug fishing village of Wellfleet where my parents, years ago, had walked hand-in-hand at the harbor. He would have been pleased, knowing that he lay in state wearing his Yankees cap, an act of respect, thanks to my brother Andy. My mom just kept staring all night, the vacant gaze of Alzheimer's. Her children and grandchildren were consoling, but her spirit was far away; she was preparing for a trip to Pluto and beyond.

On the day of my dad's funeral, the January weather was howling, emblematic of my parents' blustery fight for survival. The shrill wailing of the Irish bagpipes split the stillness of St. Joan of Arc Church in Orleans, and resonated the isolation of County Clare. In my eulogy, I quoted Shakespeare, a depiction in *Hamlet* that captured my father in a universal way: "He was a man. Take him for all in all. We shall not look upon his like again."

At Evergreen Cemetery in Eastham, he was buried with military honors, as my mother slipped deeper into an abyss. She never left the car, just stared out the window at us. In the weeks and months to come, her plummet was precipitous. Confusion intensified, the filter was shot, the rage intensified, and more and more, she was seeing and hearing things imagined. The hallucinations in her final stage of Alzheimer's increased far beyond the crawling spider and insect-like creatures I've witnessed; demonic figures were reaching up at her from the floor, as if to pull her to hell.

"*They are scaring me!*" she often cried.

We tried to calm her. All siblings stepped up. My brother Paul in California called regularly to talk to her about the early years, the long-term memories of life. Tim, Maureen, Lauren, Justine, Bernadette, and Andy visited as often as possible. Deceased brothers Gerard and Martin, I had imagined, were preparing a mansion for Mom in Heaven. And my dad, I had assumed, was stocking the celestial pantry, making sure there was a Black Dog Chardonnay on ice for mom, and a six pack of Heineken and a bottle of J&B scotch for himself.

The disease marched on—a steady, almost methodical gait from the time my mother let go, finally acknowledging she was terribly sick. That's the curse of Alzheimer's in concession; no redemption from here. The terror of reality: once you know you have something, a friend once told me, you have to live up to it. It was a teaching moment. In months to come, there were many alarming incidents with my mother. My sister Bernadette was horrified on a visit in the spring of 2008 to witness my mom brushing her teeth with tanning lotion. Lauren earlier had given the lotion to her because she had remarked that my sister's legs looked so tan. Mom's teeth were gritty brown after brushing with Coppertone. Bernadette gently told her to stop it.

"But the instructions say it's for fair skinned people," Mom replied.

The disconnects worsened; my mother wasn't recognizing her children. I was braced one Saturday night with the dread of the disease. Walking into the living room, she screamed as if I were an interloper: *"Who are you? Who... are... you? Get out of my house!"* Her voice rose with each syllable.

"Mom, it's me."

"Get out of my house. GET OUT OF MY HOUSE!"

I was in shock and went immediately to the back deck to calm down, then returned minutes later to reassure her. She understood—realization in Alzheimer's that perception is ever shifting. She hugged me. I let it go.

The following week, Bernadette visited again and asked Mom if she'd like to go to the cemetery to visit my father's burial plot. Mom was reluctant at first, conflicted over Dad's innate fear of death, then she finally gave in.

"Ok, I'll go," she told Bernadette in the haze, *"but please don't tell Dad!"*

No one did.

A cemetery is the dividing line between life and death. And like my mother, I also had been putting off a visit, having difficulty confronting the reality of end of life. I awoke that Easter Sunday to a glorious early spring day, determined that I would make the trip. I stopped off first in Eastham to visit my mother. We had a good talk on the couch, an Easter blessing for me. Minutes later, my brother Andy called, and caregiver Gabriel gave the phone to my mom. They talked for a few minutes; my mother was general and rambling, but I could tell Andy was feeling pretty good about the conversation. Then Mom, without notice, asked him point blank: "Do you want to talk to Dad?"

There was a nervous pause. Mom handed me the phone; she had been calling me "Frank" and "Dad" on occasion for some time.

"You sound pretty good for a dead guy," Andy told me.

"Andrew," I replied, "today is the day of the resurrection!"

****

Cemeteries are spooky places. I hate them. But Easter seemed to take the edge off. The sky was deep blue, and a gentle breeze drifted in from the Atlantic. Salt was in the air. I had much to tell my father, regrettably things I never took the opportunity to say. I always thought there would be another day. Today was the day.

The unmarked gravesite was barren, no headstone yet, and the plot was still dirt. I was alone, so I got down on my hands and knees and started running my fingers through the dirt, deeper and deeper, from finger tips up to the wrists. I let my heart out, telling my father how much I missed him, that we were taking good care of Mom, that I was scared, and that I never had any sense of the finality of death until now. I was sobbing.

But I didn't feel the love. Something was radically wrong.

I reached for my cellphone to call Tim.

"Where's Dad buried?" I asked.

"Next to a guy named O'Rourke," Tim said.

"Right next to him?" I replied. "Sure?"

"Yeah, why do you ask?"

"Just wanted to know."

I had forgotten the location of Dad's gravesite. Slowly, I stood up, brushed the dirt off my hands and knees, and moved tentatively one step to the left, to my father's proper grave.

"Dad, as I was saying," I began.

I can imagine my father and O'Rourke belly laughing up in heaven watching the fiasco, my dad telling O'Rourke, "That's my dumbass son. He doesn't even know where I'm buried. He's blubbering over some dead guy that he doesn't even know."

****

Death has a way of swaying truth from secular life. The truth is found in a soft, honest voice inside all of us, if only we listened more. "Death where is thy sting," to quote Apostle Paul. But close to the end of my mother's life, I lost my inner ear, and began listening to others, like a wave tossed by the sea. Mom finally set me dead straight.

The siblings were at odds over whether she should stay at home in Eastham or move to a nursing home, a similar wrangle in scores of families. My sisters, yet again, wanted Mom in a nursing home, and the boys were pushing to keep her at the cottage with full-time caregiving. A nursing home, the boys felt, was a place to die. In retrospect, perhaps my sisters were right. Maureen, Lauren, Justine, and Bernadette advocated strongly for Mom to be placed in a Greenwich, Ct. facility, not far from Rye. I was finally listening and agreed to visit the facility in late April of 2008. It was a nice place, as nursing homes go—friendly, well-kept, and professional. Greenwich is a fine stately town for a woman raised on Manhattan's elite side.

"Mom would be safe here," I thought, still feeling in my

gut that it wasn't right, but emotionally spent and wanting to accommodate my sisters. I was emptied of emotion, giving in, verified that Mom was heading to Greenwich.

After I returned from Connecticut, my wife and I went to the cottage to visit my mother. Again, she was in a haze for most of the time, just gazing out the window into a dense patch of scrub oak and pine. I spoke with Mary Catherine within earshot of my mother about plans to relocate her to the Greenwich nursing home. I was still ambivalent about it, searching for the courage to pull the cord. I was speaking as if my mother wasn't in the room; I had assumed she was on Pluto. We talked on.

"Greg," my mother interrupted, breaking 15 minutes of staring silence. *"GREG,"* she shouted. *"THAT'S NOT A GOOD IDEA. IT'S JUST NOT A GOOD IDEA!"*

She looked straight at me like a mother disciplining a son. I signed on.

Mary Catherine was stunned. I was dumbfounded. But I had my answer. There would be no trip to Greenwich. Mom had spoken from deep within her soul, as those with Alzheimer's often can, if we would listen to them. She had set me straight and I was following orders from my mother.

Whether with Alzheimer's, other forms of dementia, autism, or some other brain default, the inner spirit, I believe, communicates at some level. I saw it with my mom and I saw it in my grandfather. Today, I see it with my nephew, Kenny McGeorge, a 24-year-old in Scottsdale, Ariz. who battles severe autism, with the help of selfless, loving parents, Tom and Barb. Kenny never gives up and always looks for the upside in life. Kenny and I text all the time, as he does with others, sometimes in the middle of the night. Often, I get a text from Kenny when I can't sleep and feel isolated. I realize then that I'm not alone. Kenny gets it. He's one of my best friends. He is not stupid either; he just has a disease. Brain defect and disease is not a mark of intellectual bankruptcy, but often a marker for courage and perseverance. Kenny is all of that; so was my mother.

But reality has its day and it was clear to me, over time, that my mother could no longer stay in the cottage. *Alea iacta est.* A die had been cast.

A compromise family decision was made—Mom would go to Epoch in Brewster, a caring nursing home about two miles from my house. My brother Tim was on hand for the move. But I had to deliver the news first—a one-on-one discussion with my mother, who had fought her disease to the point of submission. The exchange between us was wrenching, immediate. When I arrived at the cottage, Mom was at her usual post—sitting at the dining room table, staring deep into the woods. I've had to deliver bad news many times in my life, all of which paled in comparison to this discussion.

"Mom," I began. "Today is the day you have to leave. We're going to a new home in Brewster," I said.

She didn't budge. She was shaking. Violently. And turned away.

"Mom, do you hear me?" I said, reconnecting eye to eye. "I'm going to take you to a place closer to me. Dad wants you there. I want you there. All the kids want you there."

She kept shaking.

"Mom, look at me, please look at me."

Slowly, she turned her eyes toward me.

"Mom, I would never do anything to hurt you. I know this is difficult. We love you, but this is best for you. I promise."

She turned away.

"Mom, look at me. Do you love me? Do you trust me?"

She sighed, exhaled as if letting the air out of a balloon, releasing emotion in an exhale that seemed like an eternity.

"Yes," she said. "Yes."

She stopped shaking.

Minutes later, as I was in the back yard, speaking on the cell phone with an old friend and colleague, Mike Saint, she walked out the back door and headed to my yellow Jeep. Gabriel, the caregiver, was behind her, signaling the moment at hand. She was ready to go. We left without her bags.

On the drive to Epoch Mom noticed yellow cars in front of us and behind us.

"Look at that," she said. *"I can't believe it!"*

"Believe it, Mom," I blurted in faith.

I called Tim at the cottage; he had been gathering Mom's things, given our hasty departure. "Tim, you're not going to believe this. There are two yellow cars in front of us and two behind us. Impressive, but freaking me out!"

Within a few miles, the yellow cars peeled off, only to be replaced shortly by another escort of yellow cars. The exchange occurred, on and off, all the way to Epoch.

At the nursing home, Tim and I tried to make Mom's new room as homey as possible, hanging family photos on the walls, and bringing a few small furniture items that, hopefully, would jog her memory. We both felt sick that day, the kind of emotional pain that starts in the feet, hits the stomach in nausea, then races to the head. Purposefully, I hung a sepia tone photo of her father, "Daddy George," at the foot of her bed. He stared down in comfort right at her. The photo now hangs in my office today over my desk.

Tim's departure to Connecticut was particularly upsetting for me. My mother and I were now both alone. I returned to Epoch with my son Conor to visit with Mom and brought along a glass of Chardonnay for her and a beer for Conor and me. Within minutes, an elderly woman in a wheelchair, far into the depths dementia, raced into the room, as if she had just jump started a NASCAR race. I dubbed the woman "Mad Martha," and she was deep into Mom's personal space, and speaking nonsense. Mom, near her end, could still recognize nonsense when confronted with it.

"Get out of my house," she yelled yelled at the woman. *"GET*

OUT OF MY HOUSE!"

Martha departed in an instant.

"Dad," Conor said, "I think I'll have that beer now!"

****

Mom's stay at Epoch was brief. She had come here to die. Often, the two of us watched old black-and-white movies together in the facility's common room, filled with other men and women in late stages of dementia. The staff was incredibly caring, but the setting had all the ambiance of Ken Kesey's *One Flew Over the Cuckoo's Nest*. I was getting a first-hand look at what lay ahead.

"That's right, Mr. Martini, there is an Easter Bunny," I recalled from the movie.

Sitting with my mother one day in the common room, watching black-and-white reruns of *It's A Wonderful Life*, I whispered to her that I had to visit the men's room.

"I'll be right back," I told her quietly, worried that she would wonder where I went. "I'll be right back."

"I CAN'T BELIEVE YOU JUST SAID THAT!" Mom replied in a loud, clear voice that resonated throughout the room, and reinforced in me that she was still my mother, I was still her son, and she was still in charge. But she was connecting dots that had no relevant tangent.

"I can't believe you just told the entire room that you had to pee!"

Her reprimand was greeted with universal applause—men and women in their 80s, all fighting Alzheimer's and all regaling in an opportunity to be in charge again. Dementia cannot rob an inner spirit. I was thankful to be part of this palace revolt, hearts crying out for relevance.

Weeks later, Mom was overcome with pneumonia and carted around an oxygen tank, as my father had before her. She was frightened; her frail body was breaking down. I told her not to worry, that we'd all stick by her side. She turned to me, looked me right in the eye, and said: "Like glue! We stick together like glue."

There would be no Easter Bunny today, Mr. Martini; the following morning when I arrived, I found my mother sitting at a table staring intently at a photo of her children, taken many years ago on the back deck of the Eastham cottage. She was about done at this point, I could tell.

"Mom," I said. "You don't have to stay here. You can go home."

She stared at me.

"You can go home to Dad, to your parents, and to sons Gerard and Martin. You can go home any time you want. You're the boss! You don't have to stay here and talk to knuckleheads like me!"

My brother Tim had delivered a similar message earlier.

Mom smiled, the forgotten glance of a young mother. She sighed again, closed her eyes, and slid wistfully back into her chair.

Later that week, I got the call about 10 pm.

"You mother is not doing well," the nurse said. "She's scared. She needs you."

I raced to Epoch, about a two-mile drive on a dirt road through the woods, hitting all the potholes in my yellow Jeep from the trot of horses on this country road, rear wheels sliding left, then right as I pressed ahead. When I arrived minutes later, my mother was deep asleep. I woke her to let her know she was not alone.

"Mom, I'm here. Sorry to wake you up, but wanted you to know I'm here."

She smiled again. There was a countenance about her that said something was about to happen. She seemed more alert, more at peace. Her father, Daddy George, glancing down tenderly from the framed photo on a wall at the foot of her bed, was staring right at her. I felt his presence in the room.

I put my left hand over my mother's left hand as she lay in bed. She was so sweet at the end, much like a compliant grade school child, like the ones she had taught in school. Slowly, she put her right hand on top of my hand, as she had done four months ago on my father's deathbed. We talked, as one can on the steps of death. I waited until she fell back to sleep, then kissed her on the forehead as I prepared to leave.

Her green eyes opened wide. "Greg, where are you going?" she said in a soft voice.

Knowing in my soul what was about to happen, I sat back down, held her hand, looked into her eyes, and said, "Mom, I'm not going anywhere. We're riding this one out together … "

The time was now. As I sat there, I recalled that she had told me just weeks earlier in what were to be her last instructions: "We all have a purpose in life. Go find it!"

I had trouble in the moment finding the purpose of death. But I stayed by her side until she fell back to sleep again. Then, I kissed her on the forehead, knowing the long kiss goodbye was over.

She died hours later.

14

GROUNDHOG DAY

DEATH OBSERVED UP CLOSE IS A MUSCLE MEMORY THAT one never forgets. Memories of my mother and the reality that Alzheimer's had conquered once again washed over me, as we prepared at Nickerson Funeral Home for Mom's final trip to church. As the siblings queued up behind the black stretch limo, I told my brother Tim to pull his yellow Jeep in front of Mom's hearse, and that I'd pull my Jeep behind it.

"Mom's going to go home surrounded by angels," I said.

The funeral mass was held at Our Lady of the Cape in Brewster on primal Stony Brook Road in the old historic district, a portion of which is listed on the National Register of Historic Places. Mom would have liked that. The church, with tongue-in-groove oak ceilings bowed like the hull of a boat, is an eight-minute jog from my house. The church was filled with extended family and friends. Older sister Maureen was the first to speak:

"How did Mom do it? She did it as many other women from her generation... with a great support system that they had among themselves. So, in the end, we thought she would stay with us a little longer, but she had other plans and kept to them. Mom, in all ways, was Dad's anchor. She was the glue that held him and us together through good and bad times ... What a job!"

And it was.

"But we have to stop meeting like this." I said from the pulpit. "Two lives. Two deaths. Two funerals. Four months."

****

My mom defined motherhood in an age when worldly accomplishment was all too often the mark of achievement. Ever petite, she could bowl the siblings over—knock us right off our feet like ten pins—with the largesse of her impressive intellect, wisdom, and ceaseless love. Good love and tough love, always justified and in abundant measure, as provided by most mothers of the Greatest Generation. She could burn our corneas with a polar stare, one that penetrated deep into the soul. There were many times I was convicted by her swift, rational judgments, but redemption is a wonderful thing. You have to give redemption to get it, and my mother had infinite capacity to forgive and to teach.

In death, she was still teaching.

My mother knew that I hated flying, primarily because the airlines always lost my bags. It was a regular occurrence. Two days after her death, I was in North Carolina for my daughter's graduation from Elon, flying back hastily for the funeral. Sure enough, one of my bags was missing at T.F. Green Airport in Providence upon arrival. After a computer check, US Airways determined that the bag, tagged under another name, had been sent to Akron, Ohio. Someone at the counter had put the wrong sticker on it.

So, I had to spring for a new suit for the funeral. Mom always liked picking out my clothes; apparently, nothing in my closet had suited her taste. Still, she was calling the shots. And she knew I liked a good ending to a story.

"Now wipe that smile off your face, Mom, and please find my bag!" I challenged her from the pulpit at the end of my eulogy, hoping she would engage St. Anthony, the patron saint of the lost and found. Apparently, she had.

Hours later, when I returned from the cemetery, there was something waiting at the front door—my bag with the mislabeled sticker.

The sticker read "Brown," my mother's maiden name.

****

My dad was home. My mom was now home. And I was starting to wonder when the hourglass would be drained for me. I can't get sick, I kept telling myself in Mom's mantra. I can't stop thinking, processing; I must stay wholly engaged; I can't let go. So, just look as good as possible, my mother had told me earlier, and don't let them see you sweat.

Letting go is surrender, Mom always said, yet freeing from the numbness of stress, fear, anxiety, and the fatigue of a fight. Pluto was looking pretty damn good to me now. But I knew better; at least I thought so. The progression of this disease is unnerving, cutting, and guileful. This monster will be slayed only when we collectively understand its extensive reach, not just at the end stage of the disease, but at the start of this chaos. As the sadistic Joker, Batman's supervillain archenemy—the archetype of Alzheimer's—observed in the 2008 movie, *The Dark Night*, "Introduce a little anarchy. Upset the established order, and everything becomes chaos. I'm an agent of chaos. Oh, and you know the thing about chaos? It's fair!"

No, it's not fair. No purpose in that. *C'est la vie.*

There is purpose in a driven life, but when the purpose ends, one must reset the timer. Death has a way of liberating one from duty. I had been honorably discharged. But, what now? When my folks passed away, my son Brendan—having witnessed the toll front-line caregiving had taken on me and the family— promptly declared, "Now we have our dad back!"

The toll had been extreme on Mary Catherine and the kids. I was missing in action as a husband and father, but saw no way around it. Mary Catherine bountifully carried water for me as mother and surrogate father, buckets of it; still does, as she had for my mother. I felt conflicting obligation and guilt as resident family caregiver for my parents. I reasoned at the time that it's easier to ask for forgiveness than for permission. I asked for forgiveness.

I was back as a father, but would never be the same. I couldn't reset the timer. I couldn't even find the damn thing. The events of the past five years and a progression of symptoms had me several quarts down. I had been on high alert, and it wasn't until my discharge from service that I began to discern my present state of mind. I had awoken from a nightmare, only to find myself in the middle of one. Like wandering Pittsburgh TV weatherman Phil Connors, adeptly played by Bill Murray in the movie *Groundhog Day*, I was in a Punxsutawney time loop, trying to get it just right, walking day in and day out in the footsteps of my mother, who had cut a trail for me. I began scribbling down more notes before the thoughts escaped, emailing and texting myself often 30 or 40 times a day, as short-term memory began to disintegrate. One day after scribbling for hours in an Orleans coffee shop, a woman came up to me and asked if I was Stephen King; apparently she thought there was some resemblance.

"No," I replied, "but I'm writing about a horror story."

The plot unfolded weeks later in a car wash. My Jeep was awash in mud on a day the neurons weren't firing properly.

Entering the automated car wash, those rubber slats slapping against the windshield became, in my mind, a platoon of horrifying creatures from the movie *Alien*. I panicked and drove off the guardrails, hanging up my yellow Jeep sideways inside the car wash rails. The attendants had to swing it around. I knew the manager, who quickly sized up the situation, accepting my loss of synapse. Redemption.

"Not a problem, Mr. O'Brien," he said quietly, with disquieting realization of what had just transpired.

Those with Alzheimer's need acceptance where they are, even in the flush of a car wash gone awry. So it is with cutting a lawn. I'm just a consummate lawn guy who enjoys riding my lawn tractor, as much as my Jeep. Weeks later, while on my lawn tractor when the synapse was failing again, I got this random idea as I began cutting my lawn—an acre of overgrown bluegrass and creeping red fescue: *Why not cut my neighbor's lawn—* Brewster's town administrator, Charlie Sumner, the "mayor" of the town—just across the street? Seemed like the right thing to do. As I headed down the steep hill on Stony Hill Road into heavy traffic on Stony Brook Road, whizzing by, often at close to 50 mph, something in the deep recesses of my brain told me this was a bad idea, a very bad idea. My attention was then drawn to a neighbor's lawn through the back woods behind our house where a delicate man in his 70s was placidly cutting with a push mower. The old way. Without rational thought, I took a hard right into the scrub pines, blades aglow, cutting through the underbrush—saplings of oaks, pine, and a few maple trees. The piercing grinding echoed throughout the neighborhood. Sounded like screams of mercy. My neighbor must have thought I was Freddy Krueger from Elm Street. I never made eye contact with my elder neighbor, just trimmed his lawn in perfect parallel lines, then sharply hung a left back through the woods, the grinding of the underbush again intense. The poor man fled into his house, probably scared shitless. Four days later, he discretely delivered a hand scribbled "thank you" letter to the house, presenting it to my son Conor; hopefully, not after seeing a shrink. Got a Christmas card from him that year, as well.

Long-time friend and watchful eye, Brewster Police Chief Dick Koch, a brother to me, commanded later that he never wanted to see me driving down Stony Brook Road on my lawn tractor. His boys would pull me over. Ultimatum accepted!

****

The nights were getting longer as 2008 faded to 2009. I couldn't sleep. More and more, I was seeing frightful images, knowing intuitively that they weren't real, yet terrifying. I chose not to discuss this, mostly out of embarrassment, for fear I was losing my mind. I didn't want Mary Catherine to worry; also didn't want—out of foolish Mick Irish pride—any pity, judgment, or sympathy. And the thought of telling my children about this was anathema. Try this one on: *"Hey kids, I'm losing my mind! But don't worry, your dad can still find the fly on his jeans when he goes to the bathroom."*

Such discussion in this earlier stage would have been demeaning for me and hurtful. I was beginning to comprehend how others with Alzheimer's cope, looking inward in loneliness, rather than seeking help from others. Who could ever understand? My self-esteem was, and is, at the low-water mark.

More and more, I was not recognizing familiar faces, the rage was intensifying, short-term memory on the wane, judgment deteriorating further with an ever slowing breakdown of mind and body, personal finances in greater disarray, and I now began engaging in random emailing, calling, and texting the wrong people in a breakdown of synapse. The experts call this "confabulation," a memory disturbance, defined as the production of fabricated, distorted, or misinterpreted memories about oneself or the world, without a conscious intention to deceive. I call it Alzheimer's, a place where the brain is searching for meaning with wrong data and randomly connecting dots.

My phone skills have become equally dyslexic. My iPhone is filled to the brim with numbers, scores of them. I see a name in my contact menu I'm supposed to call, only to find out, just like faces at times, that I have dialed the wrong person, convinced it was someone else. Such is the case with emails.

The disturbing confusion with time and place persists, along with great difficulty in determining spatial relationships; my Jeep has been dented front to back, although I destroyed the evidence with recent bodywork. The social withdrawal can be intense. I had once been a poster boy for the *Animal House* fraternity, Delta Tau Chi, and now all I want to do is be alone, not quite sure of whom I've become and where I'm headed.

The reality hit home years ago in a random Boston moment, a dyslexic day, lots of confusion and rage. I had just been given a new cell phone by a client, who wanted access at all times, with a specialized mobile radio band, keeping me on a short leash. After multiple cups of coffee and a queuing up in the men's room to take a leak, I forgot about the phone's then maverick technique. My client, on the two-way radio, began squawking, "O'Brien where are you? What the hell is going on?"

I thought I was hearing voices from my pants. The guy in the urinal next to me, apparently oblivious to the technology, was equally dazed.

Voices continued to rail. *"Godamnit, O'Brien, will you answer me!"*

Perplexed about what to say, I just shrugged it off, revealing: "Oh, that's just the little man who lives in my pocket!"

The fellow raced out of the men's room, dripping along the way.

****

On February 4, 2010, a cold, penetrating night in Boston, I was driving home from a meeting in nearby Somerville, just over the Leonard P. Zakim Bunker Hill Memorial Bridge, beyond the Thomas P. "Tip" O'Neill Jr. Tunnel that runs beneath the City of Boston. The bridge, at a distance, has the appearance of the masts of a schooner, and looking up at the guy wires lighted in blue, it offered the lyrical essence that evening of Samuel Taylor Coleridge's "The Rime of the Ancient Mariner":

> *With sloping masts and dipping prow,*
> *As who pursued with yell and blow*
> *Still treads the shadow of his foe,*
> *And forward bends his head,*
> *The ship drove fast, loud roared the blast,*
> *And southward aye we fled.*

So south I fled with a dipping prow. A place as familiar to me as Nauset Marsh, not east toward the Cape, but southward aye. My brain directed me home to Rye on docile Brookdale Place, not to Brewster. Along the way on familiar highway road, the synapse misfired again; I just didn't know where I was. New territory. The lessons of my mother kicked in: don't panic, ride it out, and eventually it will come back. Finally, it did. I was now outside Providence at 1:45 am, about an hour from Boston and an hour-and-a-half ride back to Cape Cod. I realized then that I was a bridge too far from Brewster and wanted, in my mind, to return to childhood, but instead I had to stay the course, living the nightmare. Pulling into my driveway at 3:15 am, ever so quietly, so as not to wake my wife, I exhaled—a deep protracted sigh that emptied the lungs, in much the same way my mother had respired months earlier during our dining room table talk after releasing her fear of yielding to Alzheimer's.

****

Exhalation is good for the soul; the movement of air from the bronchial tubes through the airways is soothing. The thoracic diaphragm relaxes when one exhales, ridding the body of carbon dioxide, a waste product of breathing. In short, it gets the crap out. We all need to get the crap out. Such expiration, as it's also called, links the mind, heart, and soul, staying grounded in the body. We are beings with parasympathetic and autonomic nervous systems, one purposeful, the other involuntary. In exhalation, the body does what the brain says—come down!

I find myself exhaling often these days, but on bad days, the confusion lingers, like the time when I felt compelled to join a long altar line at Our Lady of the Cape down the street. I was typically late that Sunday for Mass, and my family had gone ahead of me. As I walked into church, a line had queued to the altar. I saw my family sitting in a pew to the left; they were waving at me. I knew the consecration of the Mass hadn't begun, yet my brain told me to get in line. I could see Colleen, Brendan, and Conor in slow motion shaking their heads. My wife looked the other way. My brain told me to proceed. Others in the church whom I've known for decades were staring at me. I looked to the front of the line, and noticed that most were in their late 80s. My brain again told me to stay the course. As I got closer, I realized the call to worship was for the terminally sick. Now in a panic, I tried to discern an exit strategy. Everyone was staring at me. I stayed the course. When I reached the front of the line, two priests hovered over me in compassionate prayer. One asked gently, "Son, what's wrong?"

I searched for the right words, not knowing what to say. Still in denial about early symptoms of Alzheimer's, and months before a prostate diagnosis, I blurted out, for lack of a better thing to say: "Cancer!" It was a sobering declaration.

****

"Ireland sober is Ireland stiff," wrote James Joyce, the distinguished Irish writer and poet. My family toasted the Isle of Mists with throaty zest after the Shannon-bound Aer Lingus flight finally lifted off a rain-soaked JFK runway at 10:30 pm on

Sunday, August 22, 2010 after a four-hour weather delay that featured boisterous thunder and angry bolts of lightning. It was an ill-omened start to a family pilgrimage to plumb the depths of our Irish ancestry and, in the process, rediscover one another and revel in the seven deadly sins. We skipped the wrath part: Mary Catherine with Dublin roots, and the kids—Brendan, named after the Irish abbot who, legend says, led a ragtag ban of Irish monks in a leather-hulled currrach across the Atlantic to present-day Newfoundland in search of land promised to the saints; Colleen, a diminutive of the Gaelic cailín, "girl from Old Irish"; and Conor, named after Conor Larkin, the chief protagonist from County Donegal in the classic Leon Uris novel *Trinity*. Larkin was an organizer in the late 1800s of the then fledgling Irish Republican Brotherhood in the struggle for an independent democratic republic. Conor is the namesake of the present head of the O'Brien clan, Sir Conor O'Brien, the Prince of Thomond, the 18th Baron Inchiquin, and a direct descendant of Brian Boru, the first and last king of Ireland. As for me, I have paternal and maternal roots in Dublin, Wexford, County Louth, and County Clare. I'm all over the place.

With high expectations, the Eire trip was the last time I felt in full command of fatherhood, teetering on an edge, perhaps the last time we felt fully whole as a family. In Alzheimer's, it is exhausting, grueling, trying to hold it together. I was on my "A" game, but got pulled in during the fourth inning.

The skies cleared as we landed in Shannon, crossing a cerulean blue River Shannon. The tarmac was still wet, but the heavens opened. My son Conor spotted a rainbow, a wondrous spectrum of red, orange, yellow, green, blue, indigo, and violet. "This trip is meant to be," he declared. Conor was on point. The week would bring the best swath of weather all season, as we plied the West Coast from Galway to the Ring of Kerry.

Driving was befuddling; we're a right brain family, so maneuvering on the left side was vexing—given the distracting lush green countryside, the ancient stone walls that define centuries, the serpentine narrow roads, and wacky local driving habits. Evan McHugh was correct when he wrote in *Pint-Sized Ireland*, "When the Irish want to tempt fate, they play Irish roulette. No firearms involved—they just go for a drive."

Instinctively, I took to the wheel. Bad move. I have great difficulty now with directions, spatial measurements, and just plain driving, even when maneuvering roads I have known for decades. It didn't take long for Brendan to take over after I had wiped out a long row of orange traffic cones, brushing back one of the *Garda Síochána na hÉireann*, a.k.a. the local police.

"Get out of the car!" Brendan demanded, yet another passing of the baton in my progression. "You're not driving anymore."

Sheepishly, like a guilty young kid, I assumed the shotgun position. I didn't say a word. I knew the time was upon me. We talked about it.

"We've got your back, Dad," my daughter Colleen said from the back seat.

County Clare was a homecoming. We stayed at Dromo-land Castle in Clare just outside Shannon for our last night. The castle grounds, the ancestral home of the O'Brien clan for 900 years, is now a luxury 375-acre estate. The Renaissance castle retains its old-world charm with splendid woodcarvings, stone statuaries, hand-carved paneling, brilliant oil paintings, antique furnishings, a championship golf course, and stately gardens. The reception area was majestic; the front desk had taken note of the reservation.

"Welcome home!" they greeted.

The rooms were noble, with sufficient space for a king's guard. But quickly, we were off to the bar that looked more like an ancient library than a tavern. Typically clumsy as an ox and not ready for regal prime time, I spilled a glass of good red wine in the bucolic gardens just outside, observing a turret with my daughter Colleen. Upon asking for a refill, I was told, "This one is on your ancestors!"

Later, over dinner, the family was observing the stoic floor-to-ceiling oil portraits of ancestors. "All O'Briens," our waiter told us, "are an ugly lot!" *What a dunce*, I thought. *Don't you think the castle is filled with O'Briens?*

Our final family fling was a night at Durty Nelly's in the shadows of nearby Bunratty Castle. There, we made good friends with the locals, likely for the draw of daughter Colleen. I made sure to stand close guard by her. In the meantime, Mary Catherine was having trouble finding the handle on her wine glass, dropping two of them on the ancient stone floor to raucous applause. The shattering echoed throughout. "My Gawd," one of the older locals exclaimed, "she's goin' for a foock'in hat trick!"

Saturday morning breakfast in the king's dining room before a flight home was a grounding for all of us. Seated in elegant high-back chairs at a white-linen table, in dignified style, I reached for the coffee and cream, then poured the cream all over my eggs, splashing the outer limits of the elegant white stoneware. It just seemed like the right thing to do. A pregnant moment had given birth to quintuplets. We all knew the drill.

That elephant in the room had reared its head again. Hard to deny the long tusk of reality. We talked briefly about the unmentionable, but the weight of a progressive disease can be heavy. Even in denial, on a trip to the homeland. My wife, ever stoic in protecting the kids, laughed as if to say: find the humor in this. The kids were starting to get it. The family pilgrimage to plumb the depths of our Irish ancestry just hit bedrock, hard, yet a solid foundation. That's the Irish way.

The Irish are often slow to embrace prickly realities below the surface. We can be an emotionally numb lot. Perhaps it's a survival instinct, dating back to the Viking invasion epochs ago. We generally don't talk about the ugly side of life. See no evil, hear no evil, speak no evil. We speak no evil when it comes to deeply personal, complicated matters, taking denial to soaring heights until the crash landing of a malevolent diagnosis. Still, many survivors don't want to engage. And so it is with my wife, a coping mechanism, not as evident in my children. We're all cut from different trees, more apparent to me than ever on this journey. Mary Catherine keeps me balanced in her rejection of harsh reality, often treating me, in her own fear, as if life goes on forever. It won't, but I am thankful at times for the delusion; at other times, more and more now, I prefer empathy and candid encouragement to press on. And so I checked what remained of my denial at the entrance to O'Brien castle.

We made our flight to Boston on time. As the boxy Aer Lingus craft lifted above Shannon, over the Cliffs of Moher, and headed out into the Atlantic, I kept looking back, feeling as though I had left a burden behind.

15

OUT TO THE KUIPER BELT

T HE KUIPER BELT IS AN ELLIPTICAL ICY PLANE FAR OUTSIDE the orbit of Neptune and billions of kilometers from the sun. It is a long way from Ireland's Ring of Kerry. The Kuiper Belt was formed from fragments of the Big Bang, spin-off from creation of the solar system, and is home to dwarf planets like Pluto, Haumea (named after the Hawaiian goddess of childbirth), Makemake (the god of fertility of the native people of Easter Island), trillions of anonymous objects, and the mysterious Oort Cloud, a suspected source of comets that flash about our sun. Here, deep into the cosmos, Sedna orbits—the first observed body belonging to the inner Oort Cloud. This remote expanse holds the answers to life.

Answers are impossible to discern in Alzheimer's; but the metaphors abound. The asteroids, dwarf planets, and the Oort cloud of this disease refract reality. One is left with random manifestations, successions of real-time, mind-bending warning ciphers that serve only to confuse, yet underscore the progression of a beast that attacks without forewarning.

I was seeking answers early in September 2010, on an out-of-body recce mission to the Kuiper Belt. There were none to be found among the cosmic dust. On this particularly dispiriting day, I resolved to take my life.

The drive back from New York after a client meeting on the campus of *Readers Digest* in Chappaqua was pensive, as I passed through pastoral Greenwich, Fairfield, then on to New Haven, Mystic Seaport, and points north. I was lost in thought, contemplating the vagaries of a new assignment, rewinding tranquil childhood memories in Westchester County, thinking about my family, pondering the aggregate symptoms of Alzheimer's, and brooding about a fourth prostate cancer biopsy scheduled that afternoon. Prostate biopsies are no fun; far less agonizing, to be sure, than childbirth, but stinging to the point of nausea. My imagination, maneuvering along Route 95 just outside Providence, was in overdrive. I had conjured up a beastly image of a ten-foot surgical needle with the doctor at the handle driving it to its intended delicate and private spot like a rip-roaring jackhammer. *Zap. Zap. Zap!*

I fought off the pain in past biopsies by associating the aching din with the sound of Red Sox icon David Ortiz, Big Papi, whacking a home run. The "zap, zap, zap" became a "whack, whack, whack." This was to be a championship season, I had hoped.

As I passed over the Braga Bridge where the Taunton River meets glorious Narragansett Bay, my attention was drawn east to the 11,248-foot Newport Bridge, a suspension work of art, and then on to the placid waters beyond. I felt in awe, at peace at first, followed by intimidation for what lay ahead. The scheduled biopsy was a transient distraction to escalating horrific memory loss, isolation, and loss of self. I was now deep into a pity party, questioning my future, my value, my essence.

Looking out over to the reflective beauty of Narragansett Bay, in an epiphany of conflict, I screamed out in my Jeep, *"Screw it! Just Screw it!"* I resolved to focus on my wife, kids, and work, and whatever else happens, it just happens. Screw it. I can't control the rest, I reasoned, nor could my mom. Gotta learn to walk in faith.

Moments later, I found myself smack behind a slow-moving yellow freight truck. Given an affinity for the color, I drew near, and was drawn to a large inscription on the back of the truck. It read: "You are NEEDED." Needed was in all caps, a sign perhaps of what was to come.

I felt the presence of God within. Call it what you will; perhaps it was my mother looking after me. Whatever, I felt on hallowed ground. I lingered behind for several minutes, absorbed with the message until I realized I had an appointment with a needle. So I passed the truck, and two miles up the highway, my attention was drawn to a digital sign loop at a local hotel, the kind of rotating message you often see off the highway. There was a message flashing. It read: "Thank you for all you can do!"

I was starting to get the point. About 40 minutes up the highway, as I approached the Bourne Bridge, I was back in my pity party, fretting work, family, and life itself.

"This sucks," I thought.

A car passed me on the left. It had plates with the state logo: "Live Free or Die." The vanity plate read, "SECURE."

I felt as though the Lord had taken a two-by-four across my head as I pulled into the urologist's office. Immediately, I emailed my brother-in-law, Lou, in Phoenix, and a close Kansas City extended family member Jerry Riordan about it, both strong in faith, but I would need yet another wallop.

Whack, whack, whack. Big Papi had a banner afternoon. After the biopsy, I began bleeding from those secret places, front and back, a normal flow at first for the procedure, then the floodgates opened over several hours. I called the doctor twice and was told this would pass, but the only thing passing were pints of blood. I didn't call back again; my self-absorption with pity endured. I thought I had a way out. The discharge cycle, a hemorrhage now, went on for about 24 hours, a loss of an esti-mated six pints of blood; my exit strategy, I thought, without the guilt of a more hands-on suicide. I saw no upside in the di-rection of my life, and so chose not to tell anyone about the full extent of the hemorrhaging, not even my wife.

But "nothing in creation is hidden from God's sight," as Hebrews 4:13 notes. I should have remembered that New Tes-tament verse drilled into my head as a youth.

I knew in my heart that if I fell asleep, I might never wake up, and that I didn't have the right to end it here. And so, with the family asleep and my blood count on empty, I drove myself, dizzy and disorientated, to Cape Cod Hospital about 20 miles away, testimony again to my diminished state of mind and to the grace of God. The emergency room nurse took one glance at my ashen face, sat my sorry ass into a wheelchair, and within seconds, whisked me to an emergency room cubicle.

I instructed the nurse not to call my wife. I wanted to ride this one out alone, particularly if I was heading to Pluto, as I had hoped, for the final trip. To my horror, I was directed to the same emergency cubicle where my father had been taken years ago with internal bleeding, and where my mother, tired of fighting, finally gave in to the demon Alzheimer's. In the cubicle, I bled out another two pints. The average person carries about eight to ten pints of blood; with a loss of four pints, time to call a priest, minister, or rabbi. Losing half your blood, medical experts agree, is a sure way to expire. I had lost an estimated eight pints of blood in all. I was on empty again.

"Do you know you're supposed to be dead?" a nurse asked me bluntly, trying to engage in conversation, keeping a solemn moment as light as possible, and yet discerning my motive.

"Yeah, but no one had the courtesy to tell me," I replied.

My mind was racing at the time. I thought of favorite writer Joseph Heller, author of *Catch 22*, who wrote, "He was going to live forever, or die in the attempt." I was trying to die in the attempt and was reaching for the stars, fully detached, and now fading in mind and body. Alone in my cubicle, as doctors tried to discern how to stop the bleeding, I had my come-to-Jesus moment. The light. I sensed a powerful, pure bright light at the end of a tunnel; I was at peace and hoped my mother, grandfather, dad, and brothers Gerard and Martin would be there to greet me, but in my gut, I knew this wasn't my time, not my call. I looked to the ground and saw the pool of blood on the floor, as I had witnessed years earlier with my father in a wheelchair. I cried out on the brink: "Lord, take me home, or bring me back, but please don't leave me in this place."

Within minutes, I was wheeled into a surgical unit, and doctors determined how to stop the bleeding. There would be no final trip to Pluto today. The flight had been cancelled.

For all of us, there is a cycle of birth, life, and death. And there are second chances. The human body is intent on living, in spite of what happens in illness. Cells keep multiplying, breathing is involuntary; the brain, even when teetering, directs the intention to live and create. My second chance was reinforced with another encounter with Dr. Alice Daley, the physician on call, a caring individual who had presided over my parents' end-of-life conversation. Clearly, we were in an orbital path.

"I hope, Doctor, you're not going to give me the: 'it's-ok-to-die' speech today," I said as she entered the room.

Dr. Daley smiled in a way that said I had dodged a bullet, direct to the head.

"Go, and sin no more," the nurse on duty replied. It was a sobering directive.

****

Apoplectic over news of my hospital stay, my personal physician, Dr. Conant, was far more direct the following week regarding my failed attempt to bleed to death. He scribbled in my medical record after a follow-up visit: "Discussed ambivalent feelings, re: near miss with exsanguination. Very concerned about worsening memory; he has to use maps and tricks to function daily; long discussion regarding risk factors."

Dr. Conant then took a blank piece of paper and drew a bell curve, as if I were back in the sixth grade. He placed a large "X" on the downward slope. "Here's where you are," he said, trying yet again to get my attention. "You need to back down on commitments that require high-level cognitive and judgment."

"Time is running out," he said. "Things are going to get worse. Do I have to come over to your house and declare you incompetent? If that's what it takes, I will."

The words were difficult to swallow. I love Barry like a brother, but screw him, I raged in anger. Sure he had my best interest at heart, but, you know, just screw him. Who does he think he is, a doctor or something?

"*Worse*, Barry?" I thought to myself, aping again a line from Christmas Vacation. *Take a look around you, Barry. We're at the threshold of hell!*

That afternoon I tried to cut through my angst by mowing the lawn, about an acre and a half of it. Driving my sitdown, I was still stewing over what Conant had told me earlier.

Time is running out? I repeated to myself. *Really? Yeah, well, Barry, we'll see.*

Trimming the slope behind the house, I noticed that my favorite watch, a gift from my wife, was loose on my left wrist. Within seconds, as I cut between the reedy locusts and a thick pine, the watch, to my horror, slowly slipped off my left wrist and fell to the ground. I witnessed the cutting blade suck the watch under the mower and spit out the remains; a small section of the watch band and a silver, oval watch frame were all that was left.

"Time is running out!" The words echoed through my brain. I've kept the oval watch frame and stretch of band in the top draw of my dresser as a reminder of vulnerability.

****

I was feeling particularly vulnerable at my buddy Paul Durgin's 60th birthday party in Milton outside Boston in late spring. The town and surrounding area is filled with overachieving Irish types from Boston who have dropped their "R"s, and have learned to walk upright—surnames like Mulligan, Norton, Corcoran, Cunningham, Mulvoy, Forry, Brett, and Flynn. I'm comfortable with this lot, fully in my wheelhouse, but today I'm listing portside in the wake of more confusion, swamped by memory loss and the failure at times to recognize old friends. I used to work a room like a seasoned politican; they called me "the senator from Cape Cod"—always with a friendly hand out, piercing eye contact, a quip for all. But in the moment, I'm feeling detached and isolated, a full spin cycle from extravert to intravert—a dizzying turnabout in personality. I'm comfortable in my own skin; it's just that now I don't want anyone in there with me.

And so I made the rounds as best I could, trying to reminisce with guys I've known for more than a quarter century, following a script that I've used many times before. I've learned, as a strategy, to keep the chat short, get to the point, move on, and hope that I'm not asked to retrieve information lost. The strategy is tiring, and often "just inches for a quick getaway," as Jack Nicholson jibed in *Terms of Endearment*, I get sucked into a black hole of conversation, a gravity pull for me that is smothering. After a fretful working of the room that afternoon, I retired to a seat of comfort—outside the Durgin house, behind the wheel of my car parked on the street. I sat there for an hour and a half, just grabbing the steering wheel, trying to understand what had just happened, and hoping to drive off the face of the earth, yet I knew I was stuck in the present. How did I get to this place?

Reluctantly, I returned to the party, feeling like a time warrior. Paul and his wife, Leslie, knew the drill.

"You back from your planet yet?" asked Leslie.

"Yeah," I replied, "It was a wobbly trip!"

****

The flight back from San Francisco several months later with daughter Colleen was shaky, lots of forceful air currents rocking the US Airways flight to Boston. I was there on business, and Colleen, as she has throughout my life, was at my side. Doctors have advised me not travel alone. In between meetings, San Francisco was a blissful father-daughter bonding just months before her marriage to Matt Everett, a fine Baltimore lad with misplaced sports loyalties, at least in my silly parochial mind. But that's what I love about Matt; he presses forward against all odds.

So does Colleen. On the direct flight home from San Francisco, the airline booked me next to an Emergency Exit in the front of the cabin; Colleen in the seat next to me. The flight attendent asked if I was up to the task. *Hell, yes*, I thought. Colleen obliged. But it was not a good place for me. Some where over Chicago, I was disoriented from being on a plane for hours, and had to take a leak. Happens. My mind told me that the door to the bathroom was directly to the right, the Emergency Exit; all I had to do was to pull up the level. So I grabbed for it. Just seemed the right thing to do.

"*Daaaaaad!*" Colleen screamed in a cry that could be heard in back of the plane. "What the hell are you doing?"

With my right hand on the Emergency Exit lever, I realized from my daughter's chilling tone that this was not a good idea. And surely it wasn't. In a flash, I envisioned being sucked out of the plane with my daughter, along with rows 2 through 30. Helluva way to end a good trip; kinda puts a damper on it.

I envisioned authorities telling my wife: "Your nut of a husband decided to take a short cut home, and things didn't work out well for the rest of the passengers. That really sucks, ma'am!"

Relax. I won't sit near the Emergency Exit anymore. Promise!

****

Dr. Conant's bell curve was beginning to resonate. The bell would toll again on a business trip to Martha's Vineyard, while meeting clients at the Chowder House Tavern, elegantly appointed in oak and mahogany, near the edge of pristine Oak Bluffs harbor. With its gingerbread and camp-style architecture, Oak Bluffs is a fantasy unto itself with its network of curving narrow streets. "Carpenter's Gothic," it is called here. In the mid-1800s, the town was the site in summer of huge revivalist-Methodist camp meetings in Wesleyan Grove, named after John Wesley, the open-air preacher and founder of the Methodist movement. I was in need of big amen that night.

Looking for my clients as I entered the Chowder House—where I've eaten many times—I saw a snug anteroom to the right that I had never noticed before. It was decorated much the same as the restaurant, with people sitting around the bar seeming to have fun. They were waving at me. I looked closer and saw my clients at a table in the corner. I waved back, trying to determine how to enter the room. I couldn't find the door. I knocked on the window, beckoning the clients to come get me. They started laughing. I knocked again. They waved back, almost taunting me. I kept searching for the door, and in frustration, worked my way to the men's room, thinking there might be access there. No luck. When I returned to the window, the clients were still waving and laughing. I knocked again, then my attention was drawn over my right shoulder. I was stunned at what I saw. My clients were sitting right behind me. I had been looking into a mirror, in the moment peering into infinity, the gateway to a parallel universe, in the vicinity of the Kuiper Belt.

The memory is still vivid. If you squint, you can see Pluto and beyond from the Vineyard.

****

"Memory is everything. Without it we are nothing," observed neuroscientist Eric Kandel, winner of the 2000 Nobel Prize for his groundbreaking research on the physiology of the brain's capacity for memory. Memory is the glue, Kandel said, that binds the mind and provides continuity. "If you want to understand the brain," his late mentor, eminent neurologist Harry Grundfest, counseled him, "you're going to have to take a reductionist approach, one cell at a time."

Cell by cell, Kandel took the brain apart. Had he dug a bit deeper, he might have found that memory isn't all that it's cracked up to be. While memory offers delineating context and perspective, it doesn't define us. Definition is found in the spirit, in the soul, but one must dig for it. "An unexamined life," Socrates once said, "is not one worth living."

I was in a circumspect mood on the way with Mary Catherine to snug Camden, Maine to celebrate her 61st birthday in late August 2013, stopping off for the night in Portland, a maritime city set on a hill downwind from the Atlantic. Early the next morning, outside the red brick Portland Regency Hotel, the seagulls were dive bombing the downtown in a mock scene from Alfred Hitchcock's masterpiece, *The Birds.* The sun was bright at 6 am, lighting up the cobblestone streets; the air was crisp with a hint of fall on this pure, idyllic morning. Even the *Portland Press Herald* breathed of innocence. Its lead headline on the local and state page reports, "Dunkin' Donuts Tries New Paper Cup."

It's a story about new paper cups designed to mimic plastic foam by keeping the coffee warm in the cup, "cool on the outside." I was feeling cool on the inside this morning, as I looked about me and began to drift, caught again in a time travel. Soft music from the Regency lobby drifted outside to a nearby park bench where I sat with my back to the sea. Oldies were playing. I heard the Lennon/McCartney song, *Yesterday*, and was drawn to it.

Yesterday, I was flush with hope; today, I'm adrift in thoughts and images I can't seem to control. They rule me. Often, I just go with the flow. I've acquired a few techniques along the way. One of them is to learn from nature.

You can smell the sea on the road outside Camden. West Penobscot Bay with the secluded archipelago Fox Islands in the distance at the edge of the Gulf of Maine frames a swath of blue that runs endlessly in a way to make one think the world is flat. The archipelago, with its jewels Vinal Haven and Hurricane Island, was first inhabited in 3300 BC by Native Americans called "The Red People." The rocky coast of Camden and neighboring Rockport, an artistic, cerebral town of about 3,000, if you count the living and the dead, is a place of mind-numbing perspective. Nature overwhelms here, bringing one to the realization of being surrounded by something much larger than one's essence. There is great security in knowing this, even more for those with Alzheimer's.

Sitting by myself on a porch in Rockport with white columns, mahogany railings, and 180-degree views of the bay, I come to understand that I'm not alone. This classic Maine cottage, owned by my brother-in-law, Charlie Henderson, a retired Chicago money manager, stretches the definition of cottage with its 6,000 square feet of Down East elegance. It seems to me more of a biblical ark—300-cubits long, 50 wide, and 30 high—than a home. As I look out over a remnant of the world's animals, I spot the graceful flight of two ospreys. The majestic sea hawks, weighing about four pounds, with wing spans up to six feet, have a human element to them in instinct and in species. Ospreys are the single-living species in the animal kingdom that exist worldwide. A bird of prey, they mate for life, are nesting home bodies, tediously care for their young, and have voracious appetites: a diet of freshly caught fish. I watch the pair of ospreys practice diving runs over the bay. They fly in circles in tighter orbits, almost like the cone of a tornado, then they strike with wings tucked in an explosion at the surface of the bay. They snatch their prey with fighter-pilot visions from behind, and with sharp talons that act as fishhooks, lifting the prey to the heavens in aerodynamic flight with the fish head first. Then it's back to the nest for supper. The nest, the size of a Volkswagen bug, sits atop a spike on a 50-foot pine with a commanding view of West Penobscot Bay. My brother-in-law tells me that the nest was destroyed four years ago in a pounding nor'easter. The mating ospreys rebuilt the nest the following spring, twig by twig. The mother, he says, sat in what was left of the nest, while the father flew in building materials. She was cawing at him as if to complain, "Wrong size!"

But, like humans, the eyes and instinct for survival of ospreys are often bigger than their stomachs. The Irish poet William Butler Yeats used the wandering osprey as a symbol of sorrow in his 1889 work, *The Wanderings of Oisin and Other Poems*. At times, its prey is so heavy that the osprey can't lift it. Their fish hook talons can't release, and they are pulled to the sea and drown.

Nature has taught me legions today. Even in death, survival is ever pursued.

****

Back on the Cape, days later at the end of a frenetic summer, I sit in my office with my collection of memories, and the sounds of silence are everywhere. Lessons of the journey invite the stillness. I've come now to understand that Alzheimer's is not about the past—the successes, the accolades, the accomplishments. They offer only context and are worthless on places like Pluto. Alzheimer's is about the present and the struggle, the scrappy brawl, the fight to live with a disease. It's being in the present, the relationships, the experiences, which is the core of life, the courage to live in the soul. It doesn't matter much to me anymore that I don't remember names or faces, that memory is a lost art, and that I must employ improvisations daily, the tricks of spontaneous intervention. I am always intervening on my own behalf, just to steady the boat—trimming the sails, looking for the *terra firma* of life, simply to discern where I am. Only to find that a higher power is at the tiller.

All too often, those with the disease have become voiceless, locked in their own insecurities and symptoms, and misunderstood by those who just don't want to go there. Like every man and woman, these time travelers in disease need guidance, acceptance, trust, and love. So, go there with them at times to Pluto, try to fathom their journey. It's not such a bad place. We can all get to Pluto; it's just that some of us are not coming back.

In a stretch, Alzheimer's is a form of cognitive dissonance. In a state of dissonance, individuals often feel "disequilibrium," frustration, dread, guilt, anger, embarrassment, anxiety. And so it is with Alzheimer's. All at once. Perhaps one might understand the denial, the deflection of Alzheimer's: like the ceramic elephant from Santa Fe in my office.

Within weeks of my return, the herd was thundering again in a series of chilling manifestations.

****

The elephant emerged again today with sad words that a close college buddy from the University of Arizona, Pat Calihan, had died of dementia. A Phoenix native, Pat excelled in sports, friendship, and in life. He was an Irish storyteller, a mentor to many, a man with a tenacious work ethic and steadfast integrity. We shared many good times over the years on the playing fields, on the ski slopes of the Mogollon Rim, and in the pubs—talking about life, death, and all that happens in between. Pat was an everyman, with an innate ability to connect with people. A handsome dude, who in his youth had sunny blond hair and eyes the color of soldier blue; Pat had game. In college, we gave him the enduring nickname of "Whetto," and for reasons of political correctness, I won't disclose why. But the tag stuck, as his zest for life ever deepened.

Years ago, Pat intuitively knew something was wrong and tried to deflect it. Others close to him observed it, as well. The neurons weren't firing right, but still Pat fought on. In time, the diagnosis came like a death notice: an accelerated form of dementia. Pat, still "Whetto" in spirit, began to fade. He never gave up the will to live, until life itself snatched the will from him. As his obituary noted: "Pat was stricken in the prime of life with an ailment that eventually took away his cognitive abilities but never his thirst for life. But not his soul, not his being; never complaining, never compromising."

The end came after years in a nursing home. There were no ribbons, no television commentaries, no callouts. I heard about Pat's passing from my wife over Sunday coffee on the back deck. She had just received an email. Word of Pat's death took time to work through my neurons, trying to grasp what just had happened. I had lost a close friend that day, a brother in early life. His unwavering, loving wife, Becky, his children, his loyal brothers, and family at large, have lost a great champion.

How many more, I wondered? Too many, it turns out.

A month later, I lost another friend to Alzheimer's, a man named Hilly. I had visited him periodically to buck him up. His caregiver, a childhood friend, told me that Hilly, in his final days, couldn't discern the difference between breathing and eating. So, he gave up on both. The news—the stark image of it—still stuns today. I didn't sleep all night.

When will the escalating deaths from Alzheimer's be enough to turn the tide for more research and a public outcry to make this monster stop? The time is now.

****

I haven't shaken the news, but instead have seized the blessing that Pat and Hilly, like my mother, are free now. The realization has been comforting, though disorienting in a series of aftershocks, like ghosts of past, present, and future in Charles Dickens' *Christmas Carol.*

The night after Hilly's death, I had a dream, still imbedded in my mind. In the dream, I had moved to a new house. My wife took me there, and at first I thought I was back in Arizona. I wondered how she had ever convinced me to leave the East Coast, then I realized that I wasn't in Arizona. The landscape was green, pastoral with rolling verdant hills like the fields of Vermont, Maine, or Ireland—special places to me—tall oak trees, some hedges, blue skies. I worried how we ever got a mortgage for this mansion-like old stone home, given I have no bank credit. I ask Mary Catherine about it, and she told me that a caring friend had worked it all out. Not to worry. The house was rambling, and I talked to her about its great potential. Surprisingly, I was content here; it felt like home.

I then looked to the front yard—a wide swath of green grass, dotted with marble and granite tablets. I realized then to my surprise, I'm living in a cemetery, but I was fine with it. No fears, just peace. I then took a walk by myself, down a path on the right side of the house, surrounded by the most dense forest I had ever seen. I realized in the moment that I wasn't in a temporal place. It had the of feel of Lewis Carroll's *Looking Glass*; the birds, the animals, and insects all talked, similar, at times, to hallucinations I've experienced in Alzheimer's. I engaged them. These were not demonic figures, and I enjoyed the conversation. Fully relishing it.

I returned to the house, entering through the side yard. I was amazed at the number of tombstones I saw along the way and in front of me. Rows and rows of them, perfectly arranged. As I walked toward the front door of the stone house, I touched one of the tombstones in full confidence, patting it on the side and on top, saying to myself: *I'm good with this.*

When I returned to the house, my wife was gone. I was by myself. Then I woke up.

****

Days later, I told my friend Dr. Conant, of the dream. We talked about it over coffee on his back deck overlooking Cape Cod Bay early on a Sunday morning in late summer, as a gentle southeast wind slapped the surf against the shoreline. The color of the bay was as blue as the autumnal equinox sky. After small talk of baseball and football, Barry and I moved to more pressing matters.

Barry now is fighting pancreatic cancer, and we spend much time together in deep discussion of life and death. He has a five-percent survival rate, although I keep reminding him that, ultimately, we all have a zero survival rate. I have manly love for Barry. While our perspectives are diverse in places, we meet at the tangent of friendship and caring, as all friends should, talking about the joy of being free of a disease, yet accepting what lies beyond. I've learned, over the years, that truth is a matter of perspective. We'll all find out one day who's right.

I tell Barry the story of my crusty country editor and mentor Malcolm Hobbs, who, many years ago, had wrestled with death. Toward the end, Malcolm told me that he wished he had a faith, that he was afraid of dying. As a rube 27-year-old, I told him that it was never too late to embrace a faith. Malcolm, a Renaissance man and an accomplished sailor, was the embodiment of an intellect that I sought dutifully. On his deathbed overlooking Arey's Pond in South Orleans, he told me of a dream of being swamped in a boat and reaching out for a secure hand. I told him to keep reaching out. The following morning, he said he had reached for the Universe and found a power far more commanding than he. Call it what you want, but Malcolm was at peace. The next day, as he was looking out over the pond on a frigid

March day with a thin coat of ice on the roiling waters, a single white dory sailed from east to west. Malcolm, his wife Gwen, and daughter, Janie, saw it in awe.

Malcolm immediately sat up in his bed.

"Malcolm," Janie said, "There's your dory. You sail it out of the river, into Pleasant Bay and out into the Atlantic; you sail that dory home."

When she turned back to her father, he was gone. Malcolm had sailed to the horizon and home.

As Barry and I look up from his deck, a single white dory is sailing gracefully across the bay. We are astounded. Barry then tells me a story about his late father, a minister, and how he relates now to his father in death as a magnificent blue heron. Within minutes, the white dory crosses the bay in front of his deck, and a resplendent blue heron sweeps across the shoreline.

Silently, we sit in awe, as we look out across the bay.

****

A week later, there is a knock at my office door. Standing in the threshold is a man in his early 40s, dressed in an old-school flowing black cassock with a Roman collar, as white as the ridge board on my house. There is a peace, almost an angelic glow, to him. He looks like Father Chuck O'Malley in *Going My Way*, played by a young Bing Crosby. I'm thinking the Lord has called me home. *Extremaunción* to go! But the man has no oils or candles.

I look closer. He looks elusively familiar, but I still can't get my bearings. He calls out my name and introduces himself. It is James Smith, a former reporter I trained 20 years ago at *The Cape Codder* and *The Register*, one of the oldest continually published weeklies in America. James is now studying to be a Catholic priest in Nebraska. Two decades ago, we were part of a Bible study after work in the newsroom; some shunned us for it.

James tells me that he has read a newspaper story about my

illness and felt compelled to visit; he also tells me that his father is dying of Alzheimer's. He has come for a purpose; clearly he has something to say. We talk about the notion of detachment, an end-life divesting of material, and intellectual possessions. Disentanglement, he counsels, results in purity of spirit. This seminarian is a student of scholar Albertus Magnus, St. Albert the Great, as he is known in parochial circles. Magnus was born in the 13th century; the German friar is considered among the world's greatest intellects. He was the mentor of the brilliant Thomas Aquinas and taught Aquinas that memory is the coin of temporal life. Dante, in his *Divine Comedy*, places Magnus and his pupil Aquinas in the class of the greatest lovers of wisdom.

Albertus, James tells me, practiced poverty of the mind when he learned late in life that he would lose his memory. There were no tests for Alzheimer's then. James reads to me from his iPad. It is an excerpt from Albertus' teachings, compiled by the late theologian Réginald Marie Garrigou-Lagrange, considered the 20th century's greatest student of Albertus and Aquinas. The excerpt is a bit dense for me, but meant to take hold. "The goods of the intellect are our knowledge, our talents ... We must learn to ignore curiosity, vain glory, useless natural eagerness ... placing ourselves at the service of God, detaching ourselves from our own lights."

James reads on from Lagrange: "Our memory inclines to see things horizontally on the line of time that flees, of which the present alone is real, between the past that is gone, and the future that is not yet ... But the chief defect of our memory is what scripture calls the proneness to forget God. Our memory, which is made to recall to us what is most important, often forgets the one thing necessary, which is above time and does not pass."

I come to realize that it's fitting to forget myself, while embracing the light from wisdom, putting on what the Philipians call the Mind of Christ. God's mind doesn't atrophy, though mine will some day, but only in body.

James leaves, and I sit alone again in silence, surrounded by memories of photos, news clips, and memorabilia from the last seven decades. But memory isn't everything, just the glue of one's life.

****

My Elmer's bottle is empty, and so in Alzheimer's, I reach daily for the paper clips of the mind, a reserve of mental fasteners to hold the dots of a thought together as the brain functions like a laptop frozen in a software pinch, displaying a disturbing rainbow-colored icon that spins at high speeds, declaring the computer is not engaged. Everything is shut down.

My brain, on this day, is not responding. The rainbow icon is spinning again. Back in my office, the imagery of my memory, I look for reinforcement in a picture of my mother on the wall; the picture of my grandfather is behind me. I think about what's to come. Dismissively, I start writing the "B-roll" of my obit in a staccato style, mimicking apocryphal obits that newspaper buddies and I used to draft over a few beers after a deadline, a style that William Randolph Hearst would relish: "Dead. That's what Greg O'Brien is today."

But today is not the day. I am caught again in the mirror of infinity—seeing the past, confused in the present, and preparing to head to Pluto, Sedna, and beyond for the final staging, at peace with revelations of the present, the security of not having to hold onto the past.

The wind has shifted again. The rusted iron cod on the weathervane at the gable end of my barn is pointing to the southwest, yet another warning of foul weather fast approaching from the nor'east. I sit alone in a high-back Elizabethan chair, the same seat occupied at my parents' dinner table on Sunday nights in Eastham. I am deep into solitary, probing thought. Inside the mind of Alzheimer's isn't such a bad place to be on this cloudy fall day. There's a clarity to it, as I await the sunrise of a new morning, secure that the sun will set at dusk, hoping to see it rise yet again, knowing one day it will not, as I drift further out into the Milky Way looking for my mother.

Epilogue:

READY, SET, *ACTION*

BY DAVID SHENK

You can't go back now. You can't un-know Greg O'Brien's fearlessness, or his family's heartache. Alzheimer's has too young a face now, and a warm, lovely cottage on Cape Cod. It has a gentle wife and three loving kids who aren't nearly ready to say goodbye to their dad. It has a story that won't ever leave you, or me ... unless we get Alzheimer's.

This is just a simple truth.

So what now? What are you going to do with this knowledge? For this Epilogue, my friend Greg asked me to address what specific action the reader can or should take. You've already opened up your heart and let Greg in—that's the most important thing. But what else can you do?

We have to stop Alzheimer's. We have to. That's why Greg wrote this book, and allowed filmmakers into his home, and why he travels around the country giving speeches, and occasionally embarrasses himself on the radio, and gets lost, and sometimes feels like an idiot. He does it because he wants us to move into action and stop this goddamned disease. Now!

We can do it. A reasonable argument could be made that Alzheimer's still exists today only because we haven't yet stepped up to fight it hard enough. Smart researchers have been at it for decades, but we've only given them a fraction of the money they need to do the job.

This is a disease that has been afflicting the elderly throughout history. Ralph Waldo Emerson had it. Jonathan Swift had it. The Greek legislator Solon wrote about it in 500 B.C. But only in recent decades, due to dramatic gains in human longevity, has Alzheimer's emerged as a true social health catastrophe. People are living longer than ever before, thanks to modern nutrition and medicine, and are thus paradoxically exposed to increasing risks of Alzheimer's.

Currently afflicting 5.5 million Americans at an annual cost of more than $200 billion, these numbers will virtually triple by 2050. The global picture is quite similar: already, 34 million people worldwide have Alzheimer's or a related dementia. If left unchecked, Alzheimer's could bankrupt health systems everywhere. You've heard it before. This is no exaggeration.

More to the point, unless you plan on dying young, there is a strong chance *you* will get it. Or your spouse. Or your best friend.

There's no shame in selfishness. We should all feel compelled to stop this disease for the most selfish of reasons.

Researchers have made great recent strides, but we are not moving fast enough. Federal research funding stands at roughly $550 million—a paltry amount considering the scope of the problem and what the U.S. government spends on other challenges of this magnitude. This is augmented by smaller, but significant private efforts. After years of getting to know the Alzheimer's research community, I have recently come to support the Cure Alzheimer's Fund (CAF), an exemplary consortium of top Alzheimer's scientists led by renowned geneticist Rudolph Tanzi, PhD of Massachusetts General Hospital and Harvard University, and connected to researchers at the Icahn School of Medicine at Mount Sinai in New York City, Washington University, University of Chicago, University of Pennsylvania, University of Southern California, Stony Brook, Stanford University, The Rockefeller University, The Johns Hopkins University School of Medicine, and many other great institutions. CAF's current annual research budget, all from private citizens like you and me, is approximately $10 million. They've already scored several important breakthroughs in genetics, diagnosis, and drug discovery. Greg and I know them well (and I assist them in educating the public). We trust them.

Here's what we should do soon, you and I. Of course, I'd like to introduce you to Greg in person. He's even more real and inspiring, and funnier. I'd also love for you to meet Dr. Tanzi. Another extraordinary person. The four of us could have a nice glass of wine and revel in life's richness and sadness.

But in the meantime, please consider playing a direct role in the fight to halt this urgent epidemic. Call your congressional representatives and let them know Alzheimer's is a priority for you and your family; that they are letting Americans down if they aren't fighting hard for more research. Also, donate a little something, or half your net worth, to the Cure Alzheimer's Fund (curealz.org)— or to any Alzheimer's research foundation you admire.

If you like to help the caregiving world, consider a donation to, or volunteering some time at, the Alzheimer's Association (alz.org). They do incredible work in every state in the U.S.

Don't do this for Greg. Do it for yourself!

(David Shenk is author of The Forgetting, *creator of the* Living with Alzheimer's *film project, and a senior advisor to the Cure Alzheimer's Fund.)*

Resources

Alzheimer's is an insidious disease that slowly unravels the mind and the self. It shakes families to the core, and forces them to adapt in smart and meaningful ways.

While scientists work feverishly to stop Alzheimer's, there is much to be done for families right now. With funding from MetLife Foundation and in partnership with Cure Alzheimer's Fund, executive producer David Shenk recruited four world-class filmmakers to produce short films, true life stories, about how individuals and families cope. Greg O'Brien and his family were the subject of a short film produced by renowned documentary producer Steve James. The film is titled, *A Place Called Pluto*, and can be viewed online at: livingwithalz.org.

Other Living With Alzheimer's filmmakers include: Oscar-winning producer Roger Ross Williams; Oscar-winning director Megan Mylan; and Emmy-winning Naomi Boak.

(This resource guide is courtesy of David Shenk and Living With Alzheimer's project.)

Learning About Alzheimer's

Disease Overview

- A Quick Look At Alzheimer's Disease: Five 'Pocket' Films to Increase Understanding of a 21st Century Epidemic
  http://aboutalz.org
- NIH —What is Alzheimer's Disease?
  http://nihseniorhealth.gov/alzheimersdisease/toc.html
- *The Forgetting*, by David Shenk
  http://www.amazon.com/The-Forgetting-Alzheimers-Portrait-Epidemic/dp/0385498381
- Alzheimer's Association — What is Alzheimer's?
  http://www.alz.org/AboutAD/WhatIsAD.asp
- Understanding Alzheimer's: A guide for families, friends, and health care providers

Statistics and Data

- Alzheimer's Disease, National Center for Health Statistics
  http://www.cdc.gov/nchs/fastats/alzheimr.htm
- Statistics About Alzheimer's Disease, Alzheimer's Association http://www.alz.org/AboutAD/statistics.asp
- The Silver Book, Alliance for Aging Research
  http://www.silverbook.org

Clinical Trials

- ADEAR Clinical Trials Database, National Institute on Aging
  http://www.nia.nih.gov/Alzheimers/ResearchInformation/ClinicalTrials/
- Clinical Trials, The Alzheimer's Information Site
  http://www.alzinfo.org/treatment/clinicaltrial/default.aspx

Latest News and Research

- Alzheimer's Association Research Center
  http://www.alz.org/Research/overview.asp
- Alzheimer's Research Forum http://www.alzforum.org/
- Updates from Cure Alzheimer's Fund
  http://www.curealz.org/news
- Key Research Findings in 2012, by Rudolph E. Tanzi, PhD
  http://www.curealz.org/message-research-consortium-chairman

Films

- *Glen Campbell...I'll Be Me*, award-winning
  documentary directed by actor-filmmaker James Keach,
  produced by Trevor Albert
- Understanding Alzheimer's: Five 'Pocket' Films,
  directed by David Shenk http://aboutalz.org
- PBS's *The Forgetting*, directed by Elizabeth Arledge
  http://www.pbs.org/theforgetting
- *Away from Her*, directed by Sarah Polley

Treatment and Prevention

Prevention

- Maintain Your Brain, Alzheimer's Association
  http://www.alz.org/maintainyourbrain/overview.asp

Treatment Options

- Alzheimer's Disease Medications Fact Sheet, National
  Institute on Aging
  http://www.nia.nih.gov/Alzheimers/Publications/
  medicationsfs.htm
- Alzheimer's Disease: Treatment Overview, WebMD
  http://www.webmd.com/content/article/71/81399.htm
- Medications for Memory Loss, Alzheimer's Association
  http://www.alz.org/AboutAD/Treatment/Standard.asp
- Alternative Treatments for Alzheimer's
  http://www.alz.org/AboutAD/Treatment/Alternative.asp

Caregiving

Caregiving Resources

- Caregiving strategies
  http://www.alzfdn.org/EducationandCare/
  strategiesforsuccess.html
- Find an in-person support group in your area
  http://www.alz.org/apps/we_can_help/support_groups.asp
- Online support groups
  http://www.alzconnected.org/discussion.aspx
- Live contact: phone, chat, or skype with a licensed
  social worker
  http://carecrossroads.org/cms/index. php?option=com_
  content&view=article&id=58&Itemid=19

Fighting Alzheimer's

Calls to Action

- Short Film: Let's Stop Alzheimer's Now
  http://vimeo.com/31089084
- "Memory Hole," *The New York Times* Op-Ed
  by David Shenk
  http://www.nytimes.com/2006/11/03/
  opinion/03shenk.html

Advocacy Organizations

- Alzheimer's Association http://www.alz.org
- Cure Alzheimer's Fund http://www.curealz.org
- Accelerate Cure/Treatments for Alzheimer's Diseases
  http://www.act-ad.org
- Alzheimer's Foundation of America (AFA)
  http://www.alzfdn.org

ABOUT THE AUTHOR

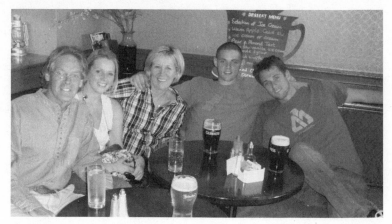

At a taverr ~~~ily D:~~~ ~~~ east of Ireland, August 2010:
(from left ~~~
son Cono~~~

Greg (
magazi
and pu
Associa
Herald
Metro,
Report
The au
17 bo
directo
Bostor
commi
on Ca
three c

616.831 O'BRIEN

O'Brien, Greg.
On Pluto

R4002203484   **SOF**

SOUTH FULTON BRANCH
Atlanta-Fulton Public Library